APHRODISIAS

CITY OF VENUS APHRODITE

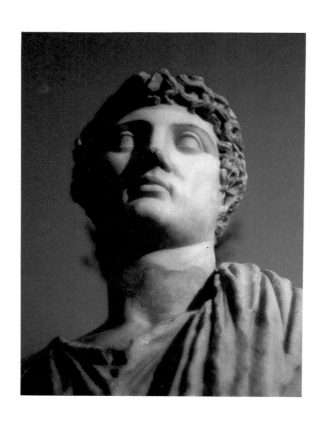

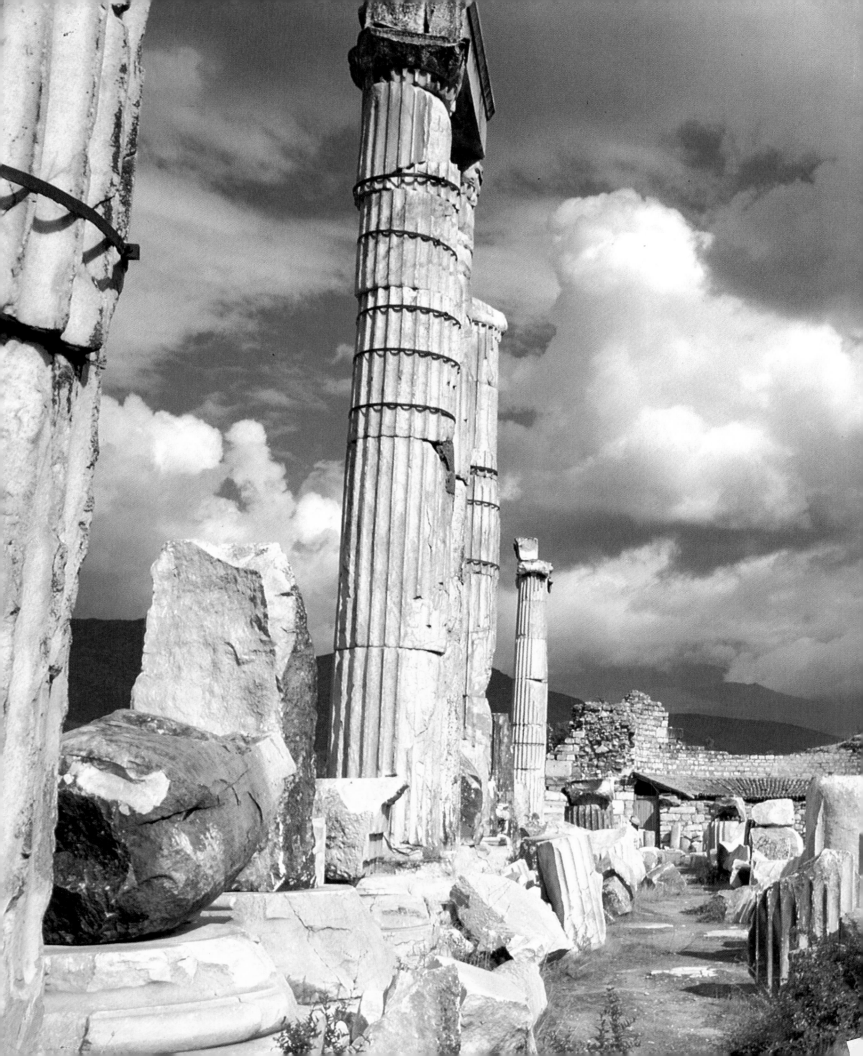

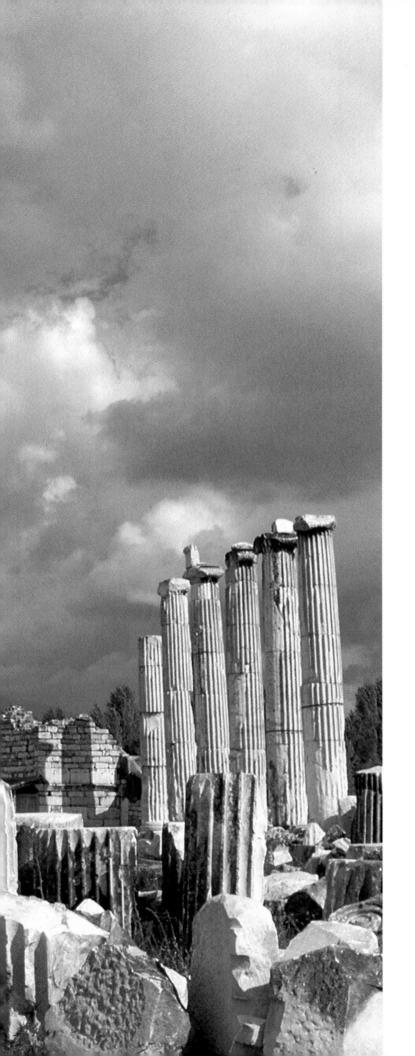

APHRODISIAS

CITY OF VENUS APHRODITE

Kenan T Erim

Introduction by
John Julius Norwich

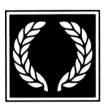

Muller, Blond & White

To the memory of my parents;
to the memories of Aphrodisias

First published in Great Britain in 1986 by
Muller, Blond & White Limited
55 Great Ormond Street
London WC1N 3HZ

British Library Cataloguing in Publication Data
Erim, Kenan
    Aphrodisias, city of Venus Aphrodite
    1. Aphrodisias (Ancient city)
    I. Title
    939'.24   DS156.A6

ISBN 0 584 11106-1

Design: Eric Drewery
Editorial and production consultants: Clark Robinson Limited, London
Printed and bound in Great Britain by
Purnell Book Production Limited
Member of the BPCC Group

Half title page
The head of a symbolic representation of the
People – *Demos* – of Aphrodisias, from the
stage decoration of the Theatre, late first
century AD.

Title page
The Temple of Aphrodite, first century BC,
which was transformed into a Christian
basilica in the later fifth century AD – looking
eastward toward the apse of the basilica, once
the favoured resting place of storks.

Contents

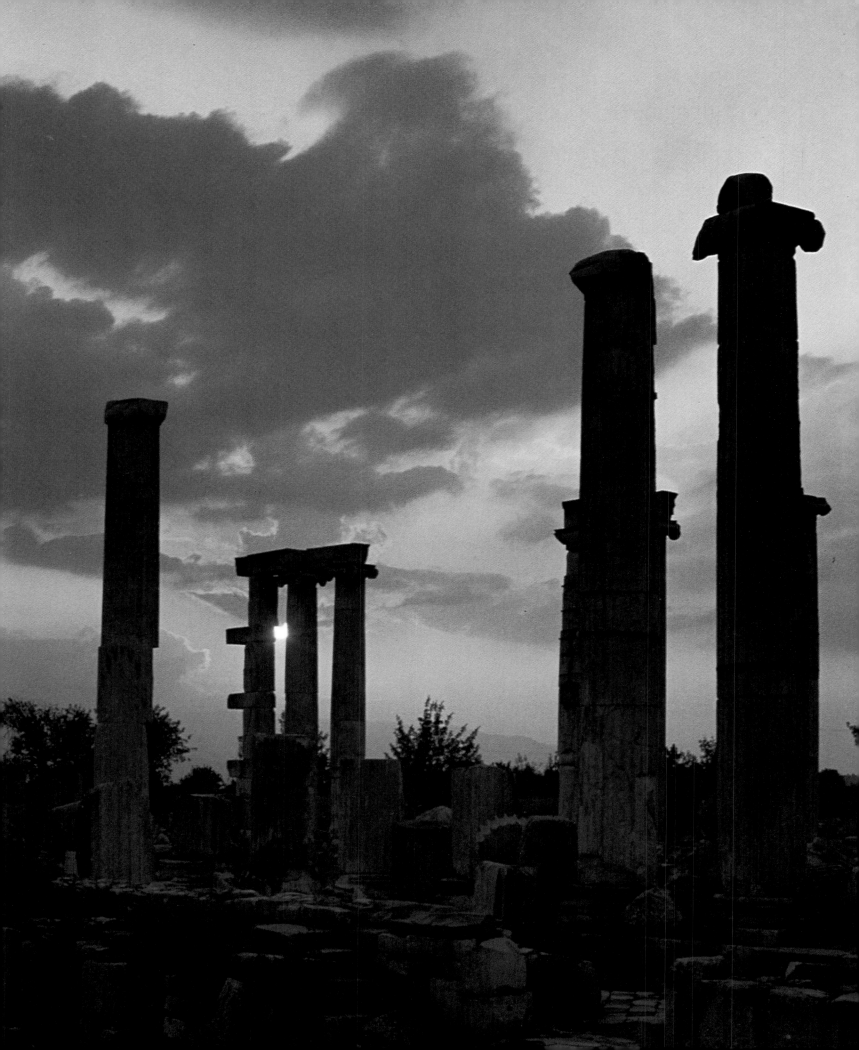

Ruins At Sunset

Aphrodisias, crown of cities,
beloved of Caesar,
laid bare is gorgeous still.
At this twelfth hour
her aged pock-marked stones
resound with life,
and let who will declare
the luck of knucklebones
for marble patrons
robed and diademed in gold
placed by the great god Helios
once more upon her beauty.
In the circle of the day
when the sun rides low,
Cybele the mother goddess
calls to Ishtar, Astarte,
and her favourite Aphrodite,
to don the purple shadowed tints
and stand again on mended thighs,
in splendour greet once more
the warrior phalanx.
She summons from low unmanned ramparts
the trumpet call of genius
to witness and assure
that when all paper words
are turned to ash
there will remain one scarred hillside
beautiful enough to last
forever.

L.G. Harvey

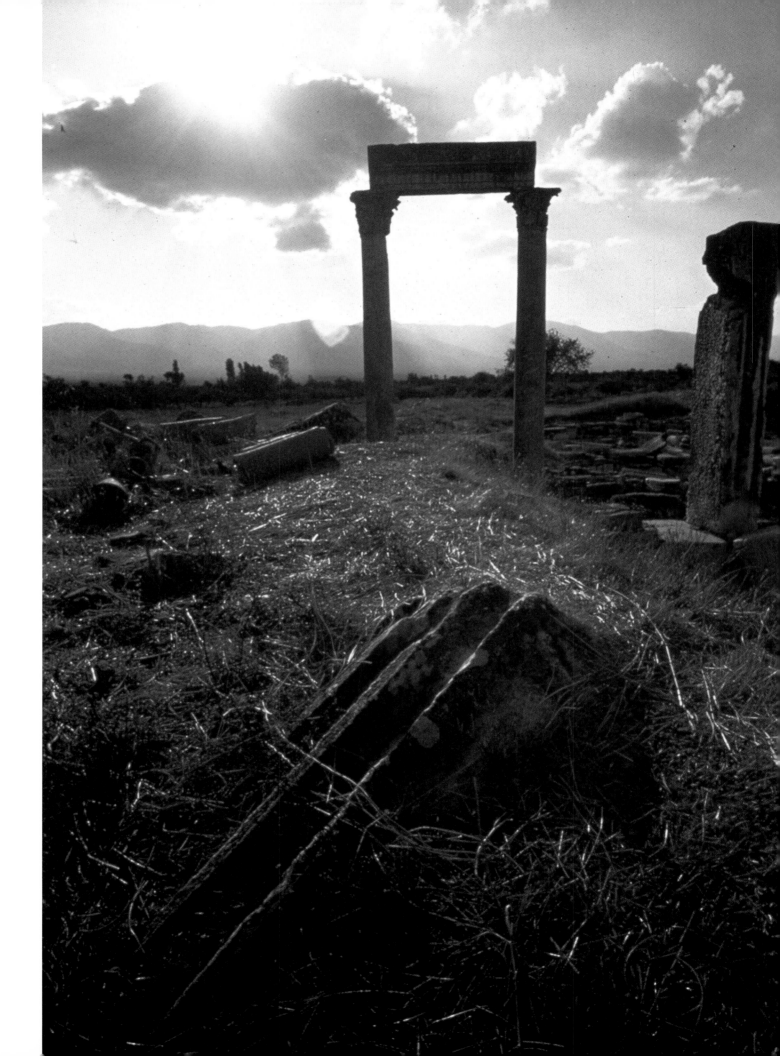

Introduction

"Aphrodisias," wrote Octavian the Triumvir a few years before he became the Emperor Augustus, "is the one city from all of Asia I have selected to be my own." This majestic testimonial is incised, in exquisite Greek lettering, high on what is known as the Archive Wall of the Theatre. It was on this wall that the Aphrodisians recorded the decrees, treaties, laws and privileges of which they were particularly proud. As one stands before it in the early morning sun — which catches the wall for only an hour or so each day, just after its rising — one feels a sudden, involuntary tremor of that same pride. Perhaps, too, there is something of the Emperor's own sentiment; for, of all the Graeco-Roman sites of Anatolia, Aphrodisias is the most hauntingly beautiful.

To the archaeologist, it is also the most rewarding. The author of this book began his excavations of the city in 1961; and in the past twenty-five seasons scarcely a week has gone by without bringing to light one treasure after another of rare and startling quality. To accommodate the growing hoard, a fine museum was opened on the site as recently as 1979. This museum, however, has long since been filled to capacity, the overflow now being stored in the compound of Professor Erim's house. I can recall few more astonishing moments than that of my arrival there, at half past four in the morning on 3 September 1984, dog-tired after a four-hour drive through the night from Izmir airport. I rang the bell, the great iron gates swung open, and there, illuminated by a couple of wan electric bulbs and the more dramatic beam of the Professor's torch, stood some thirty or forty slabs, each one of them four feet or more in height and each superbly sculptured in relief. Here was an array so abundant and, so far as I could see, of such splendour as to rob me momentarily of breath. That night I identified only Leda and the Swan with certainty; but I remember thinking, as I was led to my room, that even if Aphrodisias had nothing but those reliefs to show, my journey there would still have been worthwhile.

Next morning, when I had a chance to look at them more closely, I learned that they had all come from the Sebasteion, that vast complex devoted to the worship of the deified Roman Emperors, which

Corinthian columns of the later temenos of the Temple of Aphrodite, as they have stood since the second century AD.

Professor Erim has uncovered during the last four years in the low-lying, swampy land only a few yards away from his own house. Five years ago, that land boasted nothing but a few weed-infested ponds and a prodigious quantity of frogs, whose evening chorus threatened on occasion to drown even the strains of the Professor's indefatigable gramophone. Today, the eye is led westward down two parallel Doric colonnades, each nearly a hundred yards long, to a great ceremonial gateway with a nymphaeum, or ornamental pool, beyond. (The frogs, I am delighted to report, are still there.) Formerly, each of these colonnades carried above it two more rows of columns, the lower Ionic and the upper Corinthian, giving the effect of a three-storey building. On the two lower levels, long rows of these glorious reliefs marched down from end to end between the columns — perhaps as magnificent a processional way as could be found anywhere in the ancient world.

Wandering through the Sebasteion, and, indeed, anywhere else in Aphrodisias, one is struck again and again not only by the speed with which Professor Erim is able to uncover these tremendous monuments — and, whenever possible, to re-erect their columns — but also by the opulence of the monuments themselves and the luxuriance of their decoration. And so, repeatedly, the same question arises: what made the city so rich? How could its people afford to adorn their public and private buildings on so sumptuous a scale?

It appears there were several reasons. Firstly, their unswerving

These partially restored columns of the Tetrapylon of the later second century AD served in the early years of the excavation as an attractive setting for the everyday life of old Geyre. In the distance to the west can be seen columns of the Temple of Aphrodite.

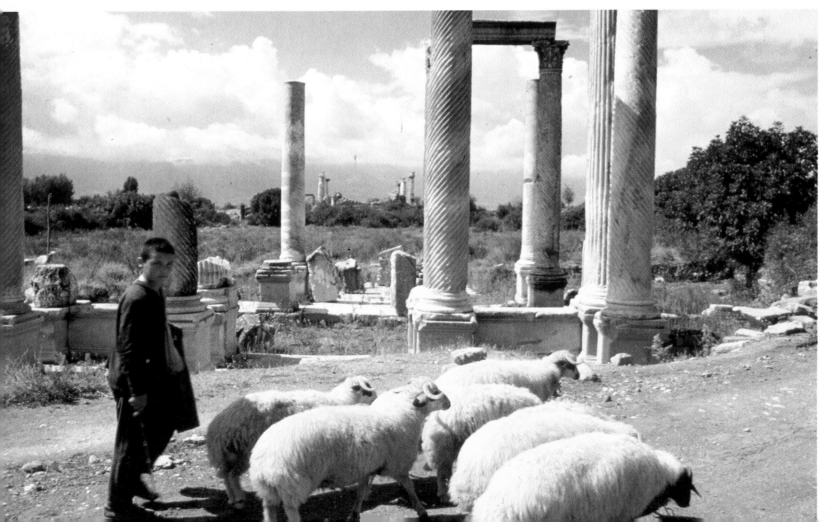

loyalty to Augustus and his successors had earned them immunity from imperial taxation — a rare and precious privilege, and one not lightly bestowed. Secondly, there was the *réclame* of the city itself, both as a place of religious pilgrimage and as a cultural and intellectual centre, to which students, scholars and literati flocked from all over Asia Minor and beyond. Thirdly — and for visitors to Aphrodisias today, perhaps the most important reason of all — there was the marble.

Now marble is essentially a limestone that has crystallized and is consequently able to take a high degree of polish. It can be found in most of the lands bordering the Mediterranean. Its quality, however, varies enormously from one quarry to another. There was also, in Roman times, the additional problem of accessibility — no mean consideration when you are dealing with a material of which a single cubic foot weighs some hundred and fifty pounds. Aphrodisias was doubly fortunate. It possessed a virtually inexhaustible supply of supremely fine marble, which was a rich, creamy white colour and sparkled with small crystals. It could be worked both in and against the grain and could be polished until it dazzled. Moreover, the city lay at the very foot of the mountain in which the miraculous stuff was to be found. The Aphrodisians took the fullest possible advantage of these twin blessings, so that their city became the centre of a school of sculpture without parallel in all antiquity — a school that flourished for an unbroken period of some six hundred years.

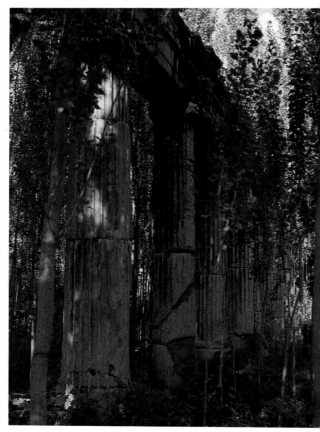

Poplar groves echo the timeless elegance of the surviving columns of the north portico of the Agora, first century AD.

I myself was lucky enough, during my last visit, to climb up to the quarries with Peter Rockwell, an American sculptor and stonemason who has lived for the past twenty-five years in Rome and whose consuming interest it is to study the methods and techniques of his ancient fellow craftsmen. That afternoon was a revelation. He pointed out to me the advantage of quarrying the western side of the rock: so that the men could work in the shade throughout the morning. They would then roll the hewn-out blocks round the corner and shape them, still in the shade, during the afternoon. But why, I asked, did these blocks have to be shaped on site? Could not the work be done far more conveniently by the sculptor in his studio? Certainly not, he replied; the only available means of transportation in those days was the ox-cart, and even though the city was a mere two or three kilometres away, it was essential to reduce the load to a minimum. Thus, for example, if a sculptor had ordered marble for a sarcophagus, the block would be hollowed out before it left the quarry. If the outside was to be decorated in the traditional manner, with medallions or masks and garlands, these too would be roughly carved in outline. The art lay in removing as much unwanted material as possible, without shaping any of the detail so finely that it risked damage on the journey.

The sun was setting when we turned back, the whole rock face — still scored by the axe-marks of nearly 2,000 years ago — glowing

In early years the storeroom-depot at Aphrodisias (*opposite*) provided unexpected and beautiful juxtapositions of fine sculptures. One can see characters from the Zoilos frieze and, in the foreground, a seated philosopher.

now like burnished gold. As we walked down the hill, Peter pointed to a high mound on our left. "Debris," he said. What I had taken to be a natural elevation in the ground was in fact a vast heap of marble chippings from the old masons' chisels, all carried in sacks to the spot by regiments of slaves — the Romans, oddly enough, had failed to invent the wheelbarrow. If that mound were ever to be excavated, he explained, it would reveal countless more technical secrets of the Aphrodisian marble industry — and, almost certainly, huge quantities of small, broken or otherwise imperfect sculptures to boot. But, with so much of Aphrodisias itself still awaiting his spade, Professor Erim can hardly be expected to devote his time — or his ever-exiguous financial resources — to the rubbish dumps from the quarries, however rewarding they might be.

For the truth is that, even with twenty-five years of outstandingly successful and productive work behind him, he still has a future programme which will keep him occupied for the rest of his active life. Four-fifths of Aphrodisias, including nearly all of its principal agora, remain unexcavated. Not surprisingly, Professor Erim still feels that his task has only just begun.

The modern archaeologist has, moreover, innumerable other responsibilities besides his actual digging. He must also study his finds, interpret them, evaluate them and publish the results. At the same time he must train, organize and control a considerable local work force, arrange for the accommodation and sustenance of his team — often (as with Aphrodisias) in places many miles from the nearest town of any importance — deal with mountains of paperwork, and keep a constantly watchful eye on the hordes of tourists that throng the site every summer. He is required, in short, to combine simultaneously the roles of excavator, conservator, scientist, detective, art historian, writer, publicist, general, innkeeper, quartermaster, civil servant, policeman and nanny.

And, alas, fund raiser. No nation in the world, least of all one with as many claims on its resources from such a rich and varied cultural heritage as Turkey's, can afford to finance indefinitely an operation as ambitious as the one Professor Erim has undertaken. That is why, having devoted half the year to his work at Aphrodisias, he spends the other half lecturing in America and Europe, teaching at New York University, and tirelessly seeking the wherewithal to support the next year's programme.

It speaks volumes for his persuasiveness that he should have succeeded so triumphantly in the past; but his work — and indeed his life, which is much the same thing — remains clouded by financial uncertainty. What proportion of his overall plan for next year will he actually be able to achieve? How many men will he be able to employ? He never knows for sure. What a sad irony it is that there should have been such immense wealth available for the building of Aphrodisias, and so tragically little with which to resurrect it today.

Of one thing, however, I am certain: his work will go on. For

The head of a Julio-Claudian princess (one of the Agrippinas) gazes out from a relief decorating the Sebasteion, built in the mid first century AD.

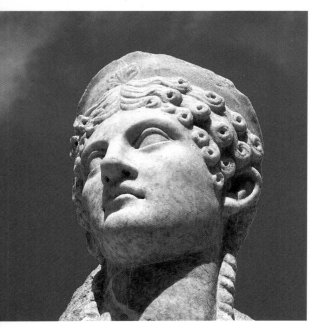

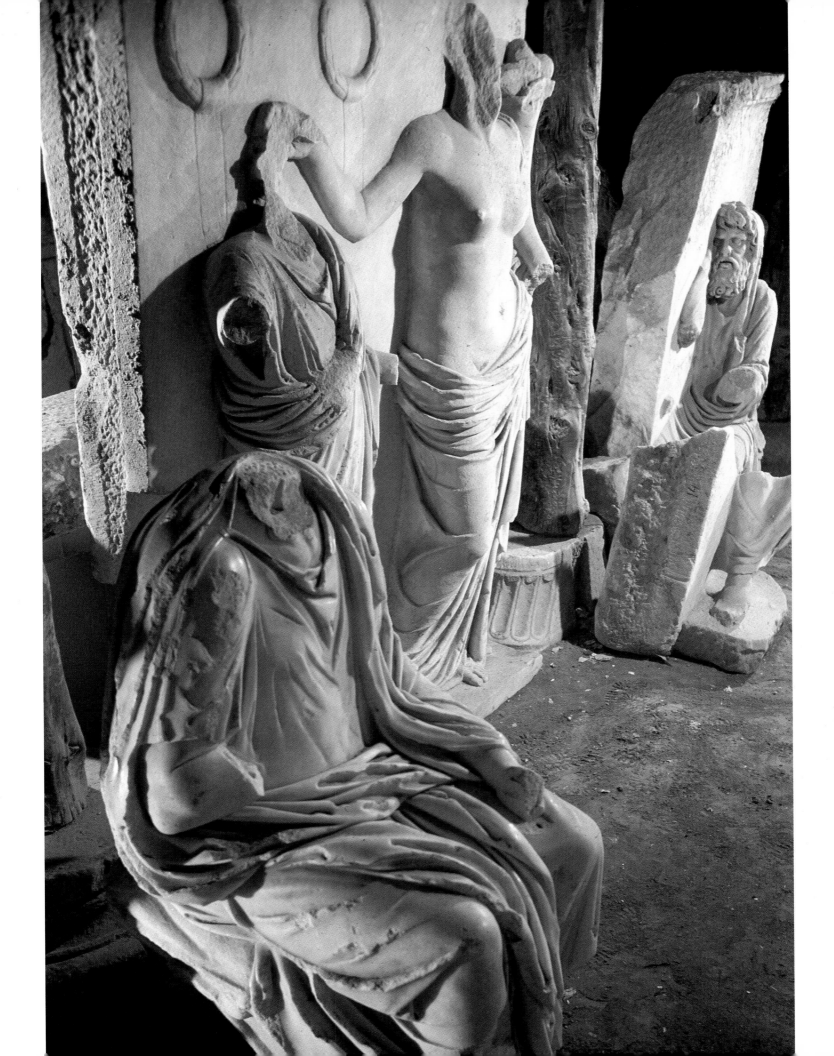

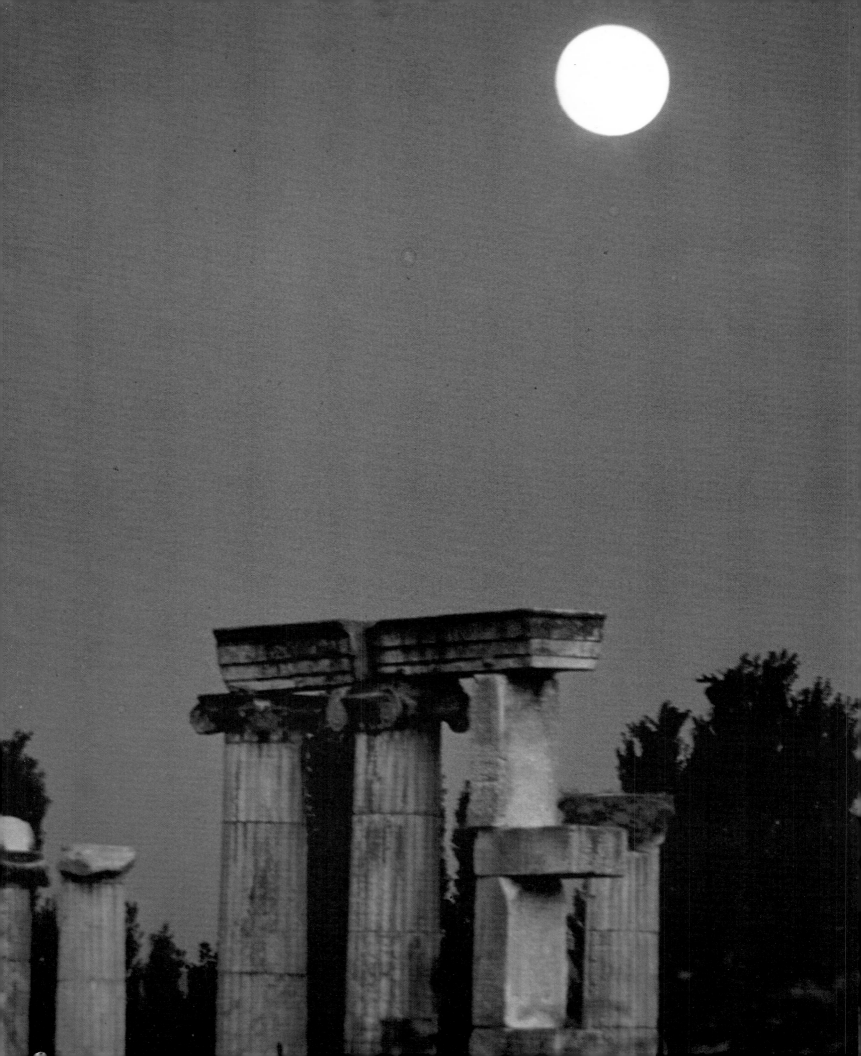

Kenan Erim loves Aphrodisias as a man might love a woman, and his commitment is total. For three days last September — and a large part of three nights — dressed in his eternal navy-blue jersey and the most magnificently patched pair of trousers I have ever seen, he led me through one after another of the monuments that he has unearthed and, by candle-light, among the statuary in the Museum, talked all the time in his faultless English, slowly, quietly, bringing the city — his city — back to life. We saw yet another sculptured slab being gently freed from the soil which had covered it for some eighteen centuries; we watched while yet another column was carefully replaced on the pedestal from which it had fallen so long ago. What a pity, I thought, that I was there simply to make a film for television. If only it had been some millionaire philanthropist who was being treated to this incredible experience instead of my poor penniless self, he would have needed no further persuasion. Those financial anxieties would be over, never to return.

It would be pointless for me to describe all that we saw during those three crowded and unforgettable days; I should in any case only be going over the ground covered, with infinitely greater knowledge and expertise, by Professor Erim himself in the pages that follow. All that it now remains for me to do is to commend his words to you; to remind you — however hard you may find it to believe — that they were written by a man for whom English is not even his second language but his third; and to emphasize once again the fact that the subject of the book is not only the most magical, the most numinous and — thanks to him — the most unspoilt of classical sites; it is also one of the richest and the most important in all Turkey. Kenan Erim, like Augustus, has chosen it for his own; already his name is linked to it as inextricably as the name of Schliemann is linked to Troy, Evans to Knossos, Woolley to Ur; and if he is allowed to continue for the next quarter-century at the same intensity as has characterized the last, his will be one of the most spectacular achievements in modern archaeology, and our debt to him immeasurable.

John Julius Norwich

Evening at the Temple of Aphrodite.

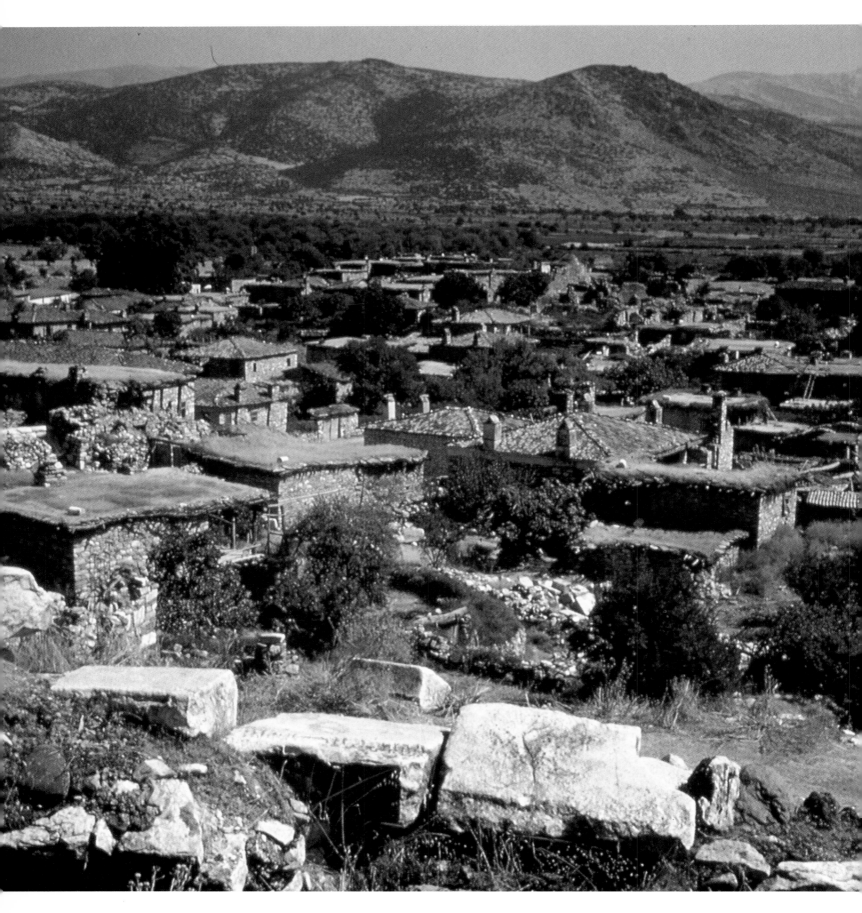

Preface

On a hot July afternoon, almost twenty-five years ago, a battered jeep station-wagon laden with luggage, equipment and a handful of enthusiastic but weary young archaeologists, made its way painstakingly through the dusty backroads of south-western Turkey. It hesitated at hairpin bends, rattled through precipitous ravines and dry stream beds, and eventually burst noisily into the sleepy square of a half-abandoned village named Geyre.

A few dogs barked, chickens fled cackling, and curious children gathered around the hot, dusty vehicle. Seated in the shade of a huge and elegant plane tree, the elderly men sipping their tea or coffee barely raised their eyes. Stretching their legs, the newcomers asked for the local *bekçi*, the watchman, who soon emerged from one of the stone cottages. Under his guidance, they began to explore the village. They were led through alleys that wound between houses framed by abundant vegetation, contorted fig trees, bright pomegranate bushes and grape-laden vines. Ancient marble fragments were embedded in the stonework of every wall, dwelling and stable.

The village of old Geyre *(opposite)* early in the programme of excavation, as seen from the top of the 'Acropolis' looking north-east.

Most of the houses of old Geyre incorporated fragments of ancient columns or used sarcophagi from the necropolis as vats or water troughs.

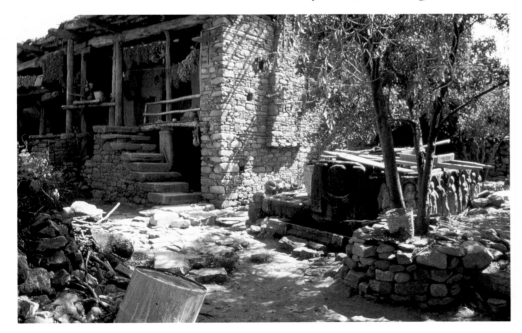

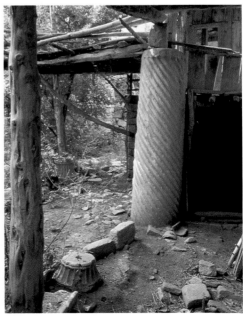

9

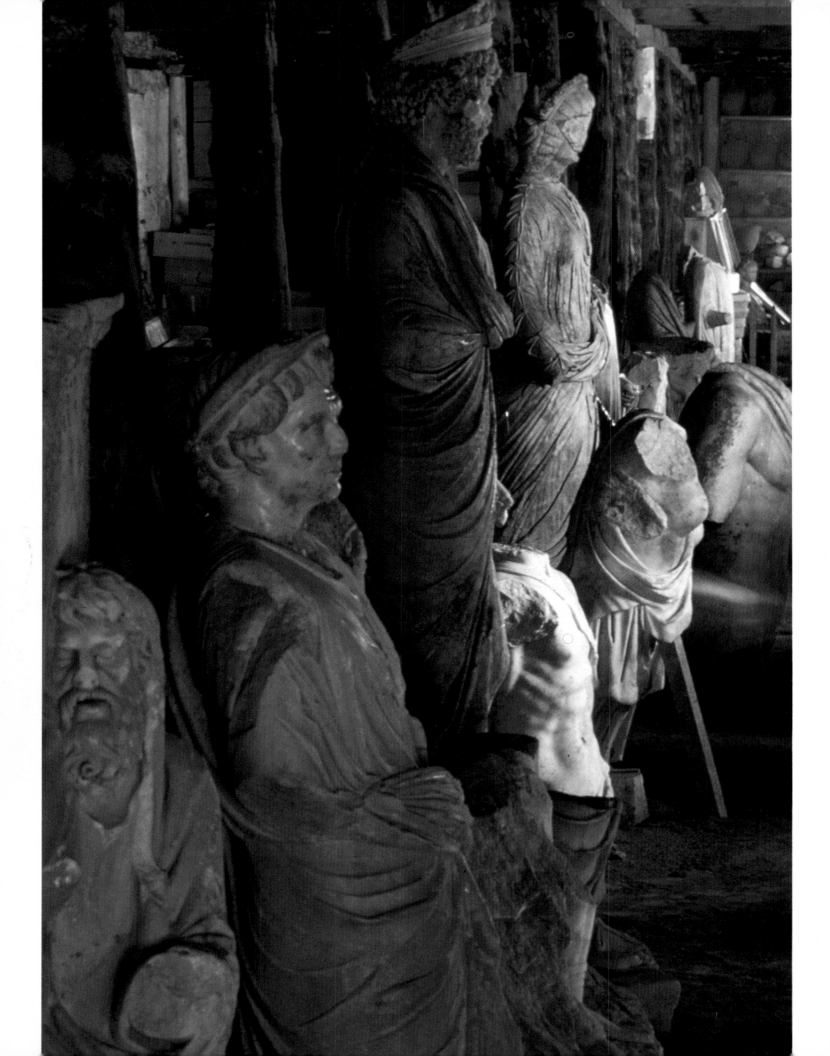

Fluted column drums propped up a stair here or a wooden balcony there. In almost every courtyard, sarcophagi boxes lay about, used as water troughs, laundry tubs or grape-pressing vats. In a dark store-room, mutilated statues and relief fragments glimmered faintly like romantic ghosts in the rays of light darting through cracked shutters.

Beyond the village houses, harvested fields and swaying poplar groves stretched out towards the shimmering, lofty mountain ranges. In the fields, the visitors were struck by a dazzling and profoundly moving sight: among the corn stalks and tobacco plants were white Ionic columns gleaming in the late afternoon sun. The visitors were spellbound. They had reached the end of their journey. It was the beginning of an extraordinary archaeological experience: for the obscure hamlet of Geyre lay over the remains of Aphrodisias, one of the most famous cities of antiquity. Archaeologists had been here before, but this was to be the first exhaustive scholarly excavation of the site.

Within a few days, the newcomers had pitched their tents temporarily in the garden of the local schoolhouse, between a tall fig and a twisted olive tree, and embarked upon the tremendous task of recording, surveying and photographing the visible remains of the ancient city where Aphrodite was once worshipped. At the start of the first excavation, an accidental discovery proved to be prophetic: a beautiful, marble woman's head virtually rolled out from the side of an irrigation trench dug by villagers. The woman was wearing a head-dress, like a crown or tiara, decorated with the shapes of towers and fortification walls: a symbolic personification of the city. It was soon joined to the breathtaking, draped body, which had been discovered by previous excavations. An inscribed fragment was also found, bearing the identifying Greek word *Polis* — The City — or, in an ancient context, the *Tyche*, or Destiny of the city. This fortuitous restoration was an auspicious beginning for this first full exploration of Aphrodisias.

The following years would yield to the astonished eyes of all concerned a fabulous wealth of archaeological discoveries of the greatest importance, as well as sculpture and monuments of exquisite beauty and quality. It was as if the spirit of Aphrodisias and its citizens had reached across the centuries, generously extending their bounties and revealing the mysteries of their past to twentieth-century archaeologists.

After only a few seasons of work, the storehouse-depot (*opposite*) situated in old Geyre was already overcrowded with remarkable statuary and full portraits of notable citizens of Aphrodisias. Additional discoveries have continued unabated through the past twenty-five years despite the restricted excavation programmes of recent seasons.

Two villagers of old Geyre preparing their field for planting near the restored columns of a basilica-type building in the southern sector of the site.

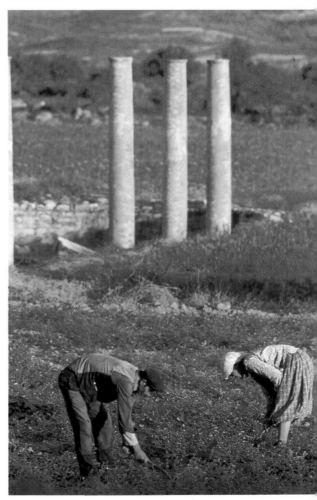

Acknowledgements

Following a short reconnaissance trip in 1959, the archaeological exploration of ancient Aphrodisias in Caria was initiated in the summer of 1961 by the undersigned under the aegis of New York University and its Department of Classics. The late Professor Jotham Johnson, then departmental chairman, gave his approval to the project, and annual summer excavation campaigns were conducted from 1961 on. The co-operation and assistance of the Directorate-General of Antiquities and Museums (Eski Eserler ve Müzeler Genel Müdürlüğü) of the Republic of Turkey, and several General and Deputy Directors and government representatives (especially Messrs. Rüstem Duyuran, Hikmet Gürçay, Burhan Tezcan, Mehmet Önder, Çetin Anlağan, Aykut Özet, and, more recently, Dr Nurettin Yardımcı) over these many years have of course been invaluable. No less precious, however, have been the funding and financial support obtained from many sources, private as well as corporate, in the United States and abroad, that made the success of our work possible. Much gratitude is due, among them, to the Old Dominion, the Andrew W. Mellon Foundations; the Charles E. Merrill Trust; the Anne S. Richardson Fund; the Robert O. Lehmann, American Express, Littauer, Wenner-Gren, Vincent Astor, Irvine and Ford Foundations; to the Department of State (of the United States) for P.L. (480) funds (in 1961-63); the American Research Institute in Turkey; Dumbarton Oaks; the National Science Foundation (through several Institutional Grants to New York University); and the National Endowment for the Humanities (through its matching grant programme in 1975, 1977 and 1979). Above all, the constant interest and generous support of the National Geographic Society, its Committee for Research and Exploration, especially the late Drs Leonard Carmichael, Melville B. Grosvenor, and Louis B. Wright, and Dr Melvin M. Payne, Dr Gilbert M. Grosvenor, Dr Edwin W. Snider and Mrs Mary G. Smith, and many others, have enabled our activities to flourish and develop into one of the most significant and fruitful classical archaeological enterprises of this century.

Like most human undertakings, an archaeological excavation must be endowed with a sense of purpose and vision, as well as with a group of dedicated collaborators, friends and well-wishers. It would be impossible to name *all* of these here. Nevertheless, it is with sincere gratitude that the loyal and dedicated labours (and faith!) of *all* who helped us to explore and study the glorious past of Aphrodisias in innumerable ways at one time or another, on or off the field, are hereby acknowledged, whether they be personal friends, achaeologists, collaborators, student-trainees, architect-draughtsmen, surveyors, conservators, photographers, analysts and technicians of all kinds, specialists, volunteer-helpers, or workmen, foremen, secretaries, printers, typesetters, designers, editors and publishers. However, among these formidable groups, a few must be singled out . . . with sincere apologies to all others too numerous to mention: Mr and Mrs A. W. Joukowsky, Mr and Mrs M. Roueché, Miss Joyce M. Reynolds, Mrs David H. Cogan, Mr and Mrs Vincent de P. Fay, Mr and Mrs A. Hanci, Professor G. W. Bowersock, Professor C. P. Jones, Mr Malcolm Wiener, Mrs Edith Isaacson and Miss Pamela Long. The present volume could not have been realized without their work, support and constant interest in the noble cause that is Aphrodisias!

Kenan T. Erim
London and Princeton, 1984-1986

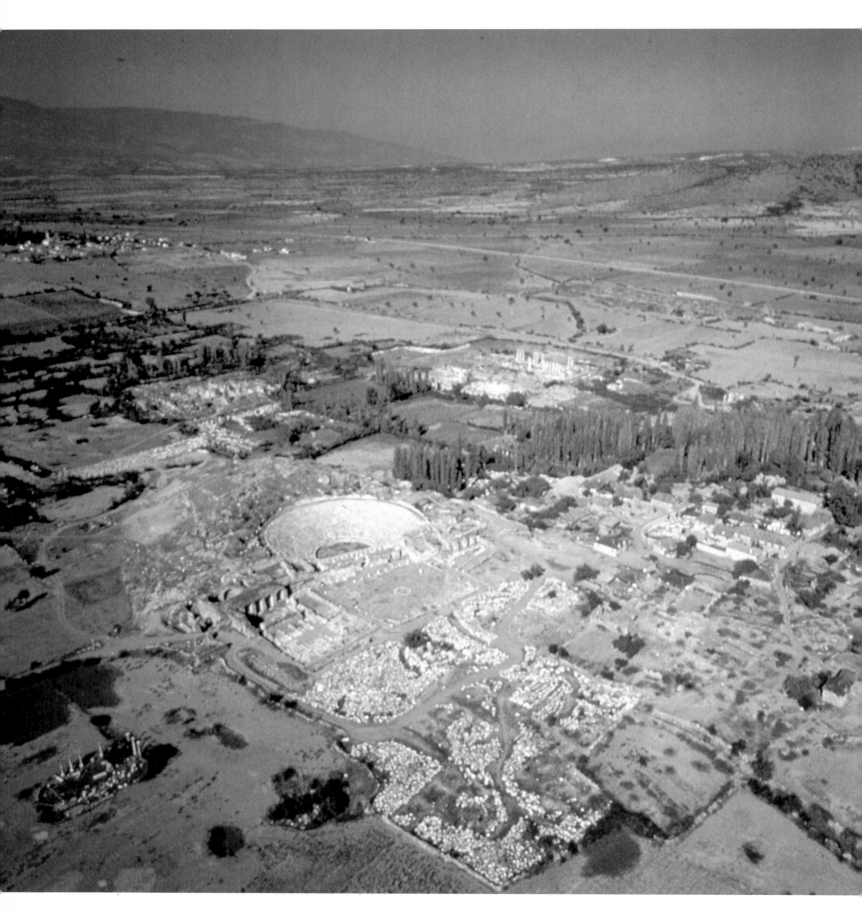

CHAPTER ONE

The Site
Its Significance and Historical Background

From the Aegean seaport of Izmir, the ancient Smyrna, roads leading toward the interior of Anatolia wind through fertile valleys and cross many rivers and streams, against a background of majestic mountain ranges. They pass also through uncountable centuries of our past. From the dim mists of prehistory this western portion of Turkey — often called Anatolia or Asia Minor in a historical context — witnessed the rise and decline of civilization upon civilization, empire upon empire, spanning thousands of years of human development and destiny.

At Hacılar, in the south-east of this region, early evidence was found of the world's first agricultural communities, dating back to the eighth millenium BC. There are also signs of the existence of fertility cults from around the same time. To the north-west, Troy was the scene of major advancements that illuminated the Bronze Age; and, although it lay outside the focus of the brilliant Hittite civilization which flourished farther to the east, this western part of the peninsula nevertheless displays significant influences from that source. Subsequently, in the Iron Age, Phrygian, Lydian, Lycian and Carian cultures marked the history of the area and interacted strongly with the influence of immigrant Greek settlers from the western Aegean who established themselves on what came to be known as the Ionian and Aeolian shores. These newcomers, although at first dominated by the culture of the Greek mainland, rapidly developed a Graeco-Anatolian civilization of their own. This was characterized by a blend of indigenous, Hellenic and oriental (near-eastern) elements, and became a rich and dominant force politically, culturally and economically between the eighth and sixth centuries BC. Miletus, Ephesus and Smyrna developed into the showplaces of Eastern Greek art, architecture and culture, as well as becoming the breeding grounds for intellectual activity. Scientists, historians and talented poets and writers — among them Homer and his followers — haunted these shores.

This prominence ended with the arrival of the Persians in 546 BC.

An aerial view of the excavation taken in 1977, looking west, shows the fully revealed Theatre against the eastern flank of the 'Acropolis mound'. In front of the Theatre stretches the later market area (Tetrastoon) and the high niches and and columns of the halls of the partly excavated Theatre Baths. Architectural fragments from these excavations, stored, numbered and recorded for further study, are visible in the foreground. The heart of the project - the excavation house and compound - can be seen just in front of the poplar groves. Beyond the Acropolis mound is the complex called the Baths of Hadrian, adjacent to the Portico of Tiberius of the Agora. The poplar groves conceal much of the rest of the Agora. Beyond these groves can be seen the Odeon, and columns of the Temple of Aphrodite. In the middle distance the Stadium is visible to the right near the road. The new village of Geyre lies in the distance, to the left.

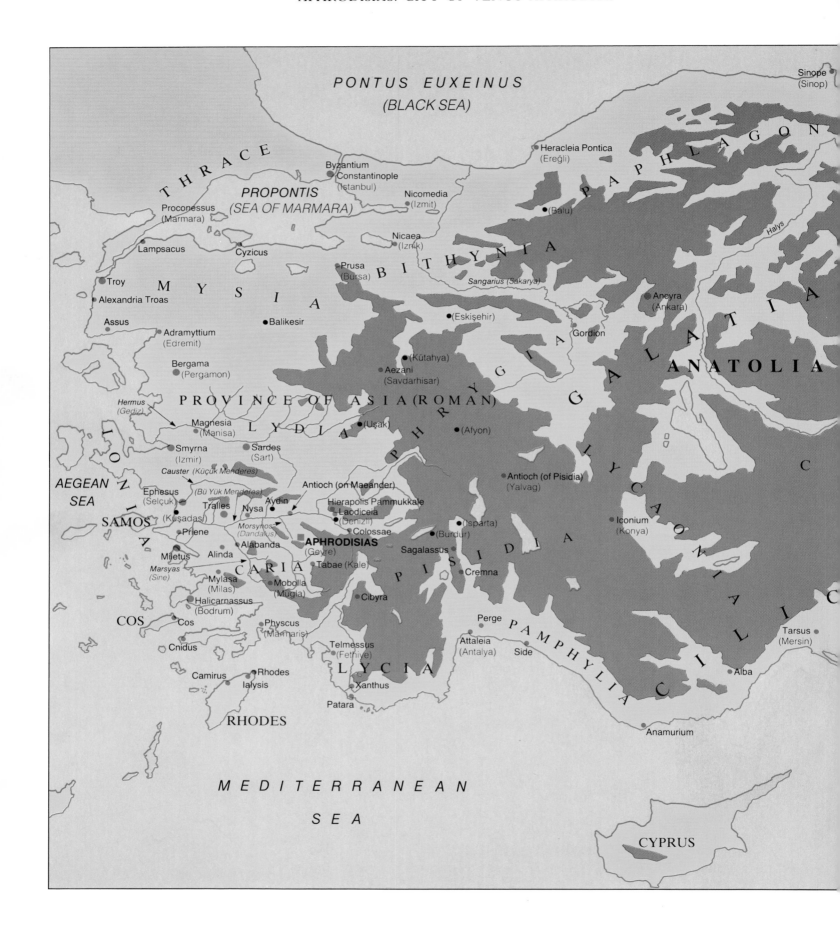

PONTUS EUXEINUS
(BLACK SEA)

Sinope
(Sinop)

THRACE

Heracleia Pontica
(Ereğli)

PAPHLAGONIA

Byzantium
Constantinople
(Istanbul)

PROPONTIS
(SEA OF MARMARA)

Nicomedia
(Izmit)

(Balu)

BITHYNIA

Proconessus
(Marmara)

Nicaea
(Iznik)

Halys

Lampsacus

Cyzicus

Prusa
(Bursa)

Sangarius (Sakarya)

Ancyra
(Ankara)

Troy

MYSIA

(Eskişehir)

Gordion

GALATIA

ANATOLIA

Alexandria Troas

Assus

Adramyttium
(Edremit)

Balikesir

(Kütahya)

PHRYGIA

Bergama
(Pergamon)

Aezani
(Savdarhisar)

PROVINCE OF ASIA (ROMAN)

Hermus
(Gediz)

LYDIA

(Uşak)

(Afyon)

LYCAONIA

Magnesia
(Manisa)

Smyrna
(Izmir)

Sardes
(Sart)

Antioch (of Pisidia)
(Yalvag)

Causter (Küçük Menderes)

IONIA

Ephesus
(Selçuk)

(Bü Yük Menderes)

Antioch (on Maeander)

Aydin

Iconium
(Konya)

SAMOS

Tralles

Nysa

Hierapolis Pammukkale

(Kuşadası)

Laodiceia
(Denizli)

Priene

Morsynos
(Dandalus)

Colossae

(Isparta)

Miletus

Alinda

Alabanda

APHRODISIAS
(Geyre)

Sagalassos

(Burdur)

PISIDIA

Marsyas
(Sine)

CARIA

Tabae (Kale)

Cremna

Mylasa
(Milas)

Mobolla
(Muğla)

Cibyra

Halicarnassus
(Bodrum)

Perge

Tarsus
(Mersin)

COS

Cos

Physcus
(Marmaris)

Telmessus
(Fethiye)

Attaleia
(Antalya)

Side

PAMPHYLIA

CILIC

Cnidus

LYCIA

Alba

Camirus

Rhodes
Ialysis

Xanthus

Patara

Anamurium

RHODES

AEGEAN
SEA

MEDITERRANEAN

SEA

CYPRUS

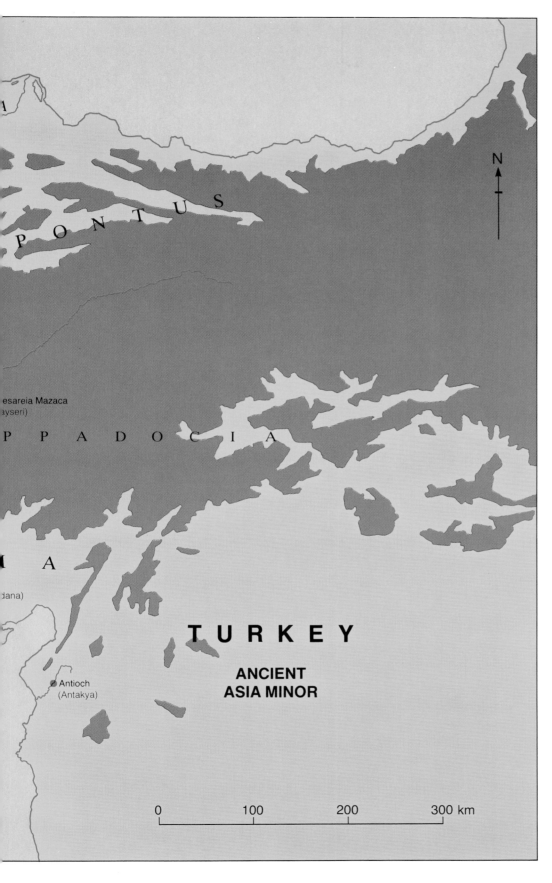

P O N T U S

esareia Mazaca
(ayseri)

P P A D O C I A

A

dana)

Antioch
(Antakya)

T U R K E Y

**ANCIENT
ASIA MINOR**

N

| 0 | 100 | 200 | 300 km |

Western Turkey, known as Western Anatolia in Roman times, included the Roman province of Asia. In a classical context the term Asia Minor is applied to the whole of what is today Turkey in Asia to distinguish this region from the greater Asian continent. The city of Aphrodisias lies inland in the south-western part of this region, known in ancient geographical terms as Caria, and can be considered part of the Maeander river valley system, which was one of the chief waterways of western Asia Minor. The Maeander flows west towards the rich Aegean coast, reaching the sea near the ancient Miletus, one of a group of seaports of which Ephesus and Smyrna are equally famous. Although the location of Aphrodisias obviously provided easier western connections, there is also abundant evidence of communication with inland and southern Asia Minor and regions beyond.

They overwhelmed first the Lydian kingdom, and then the Ionian cities: the area became no more than a minor part of their huge empire. Then, in 334 BC, Alexander the Great crossed the Dardanelles. He conquered the Persian empire and ushered in the Hellenistic age, which can be regarded as lasting from about 300 to 30 BC.

After Alexander's death in 323 BC the succession to his empire was disputed by his generals. The descendants of the most successful of these — Antigonus, Ptolemy and Seleucus — established dynasties (the so-called Antigonids, Ptolemies and Seleucids) which contended at various times for the possession of western Anatolia. Another Hellenistic dynasty, the Attalids of Pergamon, came to dominate the area in the third and second centuries BC. They founded new cities and encouraged artistic and cultural activities. Through their influence, western Asia Minor became once more a leading and influential centre of the arts in the eastern if not the whole Mediterranean region. This cultural flowering persisted even after the beginning of Roman rule in the later second century BC.

During the centuries of Roman rule, western Anatolian cities were among the most significant centres of art and culture in the empire. They continued their dominant role even after the advent of Christianity in the fourth century, the fracture of the Roman empire, and the formation of an eastern portion of it into the Byzantine empire. From the seventh century on, however plagues, natural catastrophies, economic and political ills, invasions and religious strife deeply undermined the prosperity of the once splendid cities of western Anatolia. Many of them declined in wealth and power, shrank considerably in population, or were even abandoned.

The arrival of the Seljuk Turks in the eleventh century introduced a new cultural and religious element. Despite many pressures and occasional invasions the Byzantine empire nevertheless continued to hold its own, although over a steadily diminishing area, until the fall of its capital at Constantinople in 1453 to the Ottoman Turks. Western Anatolia then became a small part of the huge Ottoman empire that stretched at one time as far as the gates of Vienna and lasted for almost five centuries until the First World War.

The ancient city that has become the present site of Aphrodisias is located two hundred and forty kilometres south-east of Izmir, at an altitude of about six hundred metres above sea-level. It is administratively tied to the *vilâyet* (province) of Aydin (ancient Tralles) and the *kaza* (county) of Karacasu.

In 1956, the area to the south-east of Aphrodisias suffered a serious earthquake. Although neither the site itself nor the village of Geyre which covered part of it were much affected, the authorities, sensing the archaeological potential of Aphrodisias and concerned about the makeshift construction of the houses of Geyre, decreed that a new village would be built about two kilometres to the west of the Byzantine fortification walls of the ancient city. Despite this decree, the construction of new Geyre proceeded slowly. The

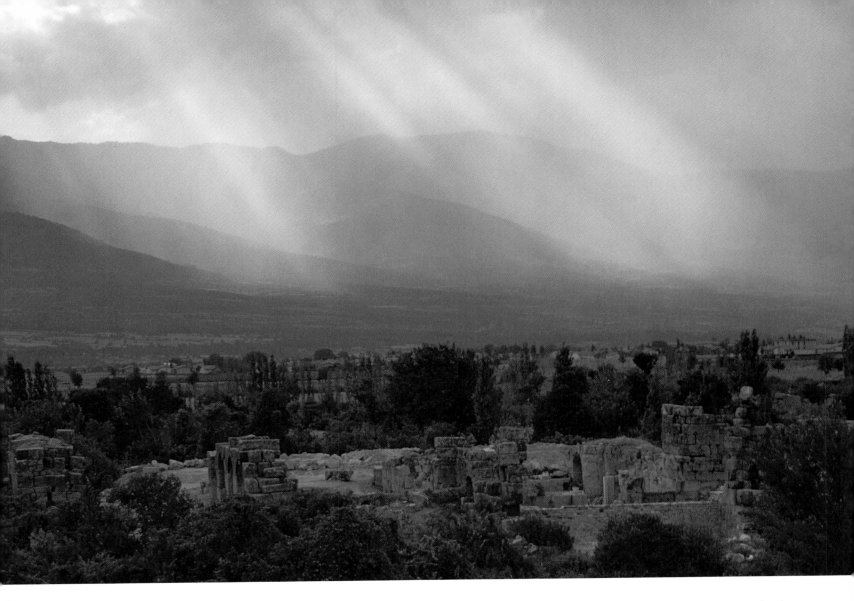

transfer of the inhabitants did not seriously begin until well after excavations commenced in 1961, although it proceeded more rapidly after the official inauguration of the Museum in 1979. Today, the greater part of old Geyre, occupying the south-eastern sector of the ancient city, as well as some of the outlying fields within the medieval fortification system, have been purchased on behalf of the project. Although the limits defining the site of Aphrodisias have been officially approved, much of the ancient city within these boundaries still remains privately owned as fields and orchards. The ultimate goal of the project must be to acquire all of these, in order to protect the site as much as possible and eventually transform it into an archaeological haven.

It is probable that in antiquity the area around Aphrodisias did not look very different from today. Abundant vegetation, orchards, vines, flowering plants and groves of trees must have filled the plateau. Then, as now, streams cascaded down the neighbouring eastern mountains and joined their waters to form the modern Dandalas, a tributary of the Maeander (the modern Menderes) which flows north-eastward. One difference must be that the slopes of Baba Dağ (the ancient Salbakos mountains) were undoubtedly

The sun's rays penetrate the gathering clouds of an approaching storm over the Karincali Dağ range to the west of Aphrodisias, providing a dramatic backdrop to the Baths of Hadrian, seen from the 'Acropolis'.

19

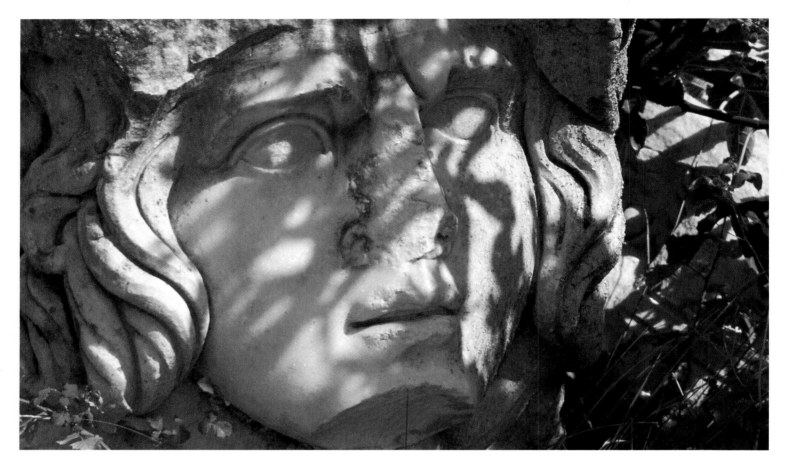

Half-hidden among the brambles, near the Baths of Hadrian, a colossal head of Medusa peers out of the shadows with a melancholy gaze.

more wooded than they are now. For, as in the rest of the Mediterranean, indiscriminate tree-felling, an absence of planned reforestation, and the ubiquitous herds of goats — the scourge of young saplings — have done much to denude them. Nevertheless, the principal assets of the site were — and still are — the fertility of its soil and the abundance of its life-giving springs. Another prerequisite for the satisfactory development of prehistoric settlements, namely the proximity of good flint sources for the fashioning of stone tools, has also been recently located in the vicinity of the Dandalas, north-west of the site.

Each of these factors was no doubt significant in attracting early man to the area and in determining the growth of prehistoric settlements. A wealth of archaeological evidence pertaining to the earliest phases of Aphrodisias' existence has been extracted from two artificial mounds, or *höyük*, situated in what became the heart of the Graeco-Roman and Byzantine city. These have revealed occupation of the area dating back to at least 5,800 BC (the late Neolithic and Chalcolithic period) and spanning most of the Bronze and Early Iron Ages.

The geographical situation of Aphrodisias must also have helped its development. It was slightly distant from, yet well connected with, the main network of roads to the north-west and the south-east. It therefore enjoyed some degree of security without being too

20

far removed from the main stream of traffic. Today, however, despite the excellent asphalt road completed by the Turkish Department of Highways in 1972, Aphrodisias still appears to be a long way from the busy Izmir-Denizli and Burdur-Antalya road systems which in part follow the Maeander valley. The process of isolation probably began with the gradual decline of the Byzantine empire and accelerated in Ottoman times. Doubtless it was further affected by the growth at that time of the *kaza* of Karacasu. Due to the latter's less exposed or vulnerable position on terraces along the slopes of the Karıncali Dağ (ancient Mesogis), Karacasu slowly drew away traffic from Aphrodisias-Geyre, as it continues to do to some extent today. In Roman, and probably pre-Roman, times Aphrodisias had been joined directly to the Maeander valley by a road (some traces of which remain) following the valley of the Dandalas and ending at ancient Antioch-on-the-Maeander (modern Başaran). When the Turkish Department of Highways planned the current link of Aphrodisias-Geyre to the Maeander valley in the 1960s, it seriously considered following the path of the ancient Roman road. Since this would have meant by-passing Karacasu, however, political pressures were brought to bear on the plan, which as a result was not carried out.

Today, as in antiquity, the road heading south-eastward from Aphrodisias leads to the higher plateau of ancient Tabae (modern Kale), across imposing mountain ranges, and on to the modern towns of Denizli, to the north, and Muğla, Elmalı and Burdur, to the south and east. Continuing south-eastward, the road leads through parts of the ancient provinces of Pisidia, Lycia and Pamphylia to the coast at Antalya. Stray archaeological evidence and limited investigations indicate that a chain of very important prehistoric sites, including Hacılar, which had cultural affinities with Aphrodisias, existed along this route.

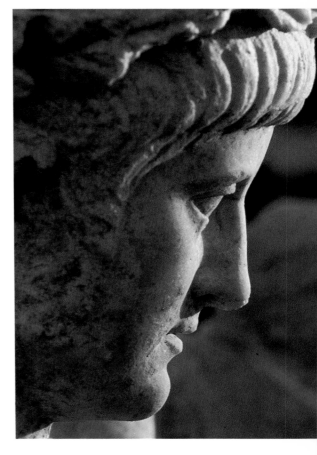

The perfect profile of a handsome Julio-Claudian prince that decorated one of the reliefs of the Sebasteion illustrates the skill of the Aphrodisian sculptors as well as the excellent condition of much of the marble recovered in the excavations.

Many ancient sites or cities bear witness to the past glories of this region's diverse and fascinating history. Today, in the hinterland of Izmir, the archaeologically inclined traveller can appreciate a compelling panorama of art, mythology and history. To the north is Troy. The name still strongly evokes the stories of the Iliad, even though the visible remains are as much a monument to that flamboyant excavator, Schliemann, as to Homer's gods and heroes. Pergamon, perched on the slopes of a steep acropolis, reflects the ruined aspiration of its Attalid dynasty, while the monuments of Sardis to the east recall an older association with the fabulous wealth of King Croesus and Midas of the golden touch. Overlooking a silted harbour to the south, the sprawling ruins of Ephesus stretch out in a dazzling extravagance of marble. Farther south still, the handsome Carian shores vividly bring to mind Mausolus and

Artemisia at Halicarnassus (modern Bodrum) and Praxiteles'
Aphrodite at Knidos, although little survives of their much admired
monuments and creations. The remains of Miletus lie forlorn in the
flat estuary plain of the Maeander where well-watered cotton fields
and thick reeds grow over its once proud porticos and lively
market-places. Farther eastward, toward the interior, along the
course of the Maeander river, the valley and mountain slopes are
arrayed with equally evocative if less well-known archaeological
sites and ancient cities, among them Alabanda, Alinda, Labranda,
Nyssa and Tralles.

High in the uplands above the Maeander, to the south-east, a
group of small tributaries of the river descends from the neighbouring ranges and, fed by abundant winter snows and rains, water a
high plateau surrounded by the ranges of the great Baba Dağ mountains. An unusual abundance of springs and underground streams
transforms the area into a veritable oasis of greenery, accentuated by
the tall, elegant silhouettes of poplar trees. Here, in this wealth of
verdant shade, at the foot of a jagged peak of the Salbakos range, lie
the remains of Aphrodisias.

Few archaeological sites — either elsewhere in Turkey or indeed
in the whole Mediterranean basin — cast as profound and magical a
spell as Aphrodisias does upon its visitor. My first experience of this
occurred in 1959 during a preliminary inspection of the region with
a view to launching the archaeological exploration of a classical site
under the aegis of New York University. Despite an extraordinarily
arduous journey, the first reaction of my colleagues and myself to
the city of Aphrodite was a pure enchantment. We were excited,
delighted and amazed as we browsed among an extraordinarily
happy blend of cultivated fields, orchards and half buried remains of
exquisitely proportioned and impressive ancient monuments that
identified the ancient city. It reinforced our already strong desire to
unravel their past history and especially our original wish to learn
more about the remarkable sculptors who were reputed to have
hailed from here. Since 1959 the magic has never stopped.

Although the organization and financing of such a project were by
no means easy tasks, the excavations were launched with a preliminary survey of the site in 1961. Work was subsequently continued in
yearly summer campaigns. Since only perfunctory investigations
had been undertaken at the site before, namely in 1904-1905 and in
1937, our work focused on the history, and prehistory, of Aphrodisias as well as on the artistic merits and activities of the talented
sculptors whose signatures had carried the name of their native city
far and wide through the Roman empire.

The results achieved in the course of twenty-five summers have
more than surpassed our initial expectations, and can be rightly
considered outstanding, if not spectacular, by any standards. Not
only have crucial data about the prehistory and history of the area
been gained, but also monuments of particular significance and

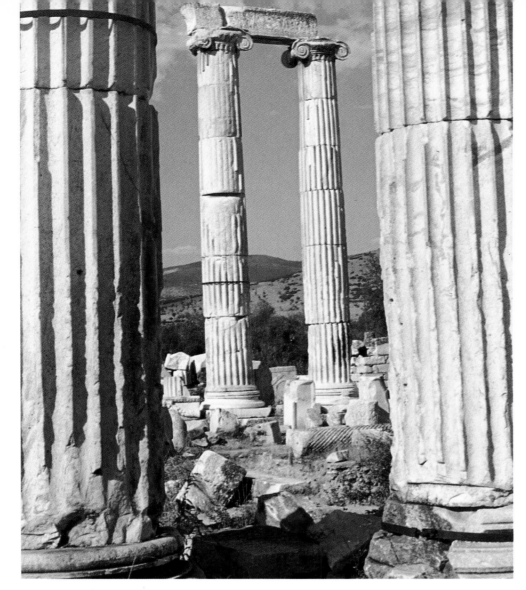

Like battered sentinels. the Ionic columns of the Temple of Aphrodite have withstood earthquake, storm and tempest for nearly 2,000 years.

beauty, often in excellent states of preservation, have been brought to light. Great quantities of archaeological material, including important inscriptions, coins, pottery, terracottas, jewellery, mosaic floors and frescos have been recorded or restored. All these are currently being studied or prepared for publication, and they will make significant and original contributions to the archaeology of Asia Minor and the ancient Mediterranean.

Especially worthy of our attention and admiration, however, are the exceptional quantity and quality of the sculptural finds. These range from reliefs to sarcophagi and altars, and include many important life-size or colossal portrait statues of Roman emperors and notables from the first five centuries AD. These, in addition to countless half-finished or trial pieces recorded everywhere at the site and the presence of excellent marble supplies in the neighbouring mountains, proved beyond doubt the existence of a highly original Aphrodisian school of sculpture that flourished from the first century BC to the late fifth and early sixth century AD. Thus the excavations have provided a most rewarding new contribution to the history of ancient art, and specifically to that of Graeco-Roman and Early Byzantine sculpture.

23

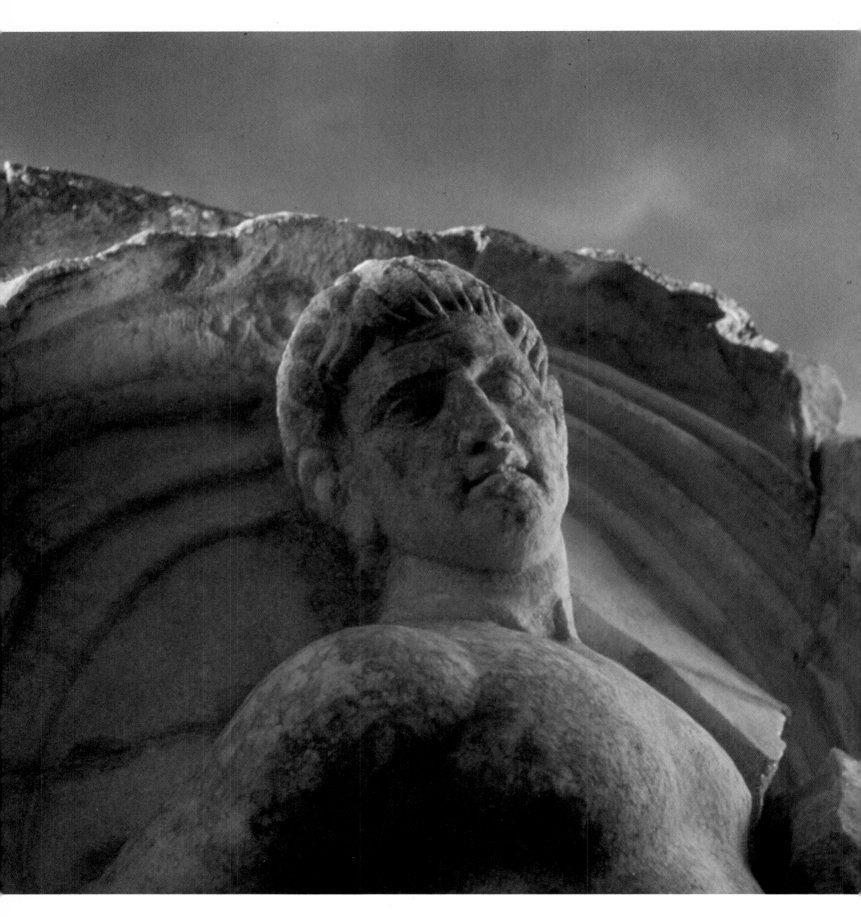

CHAPTER TWO

The History of Aphrodisias

Ancient textual references to Aphrodisias are not very numerous. This is not unusual among ancient sites, when one considers how many of the historical writings of antiquity have been lost. Nor does it mean that Aphrodisias was neither insignificant nor unimportant. In consequence, the role played by archaeology in supplementing limited written sources with physical evidence is crucial. A reconstruction of the history and prehistory of Aphrodisias can be achieved, albeit with some gaps, through a combination of the few surviving ancient references with the vast and remarkably coherent body of archaeological data uncovered over the past two decades.

According to most ancient sources, Aphrodisias was located in the north-east region of Anatolia, or Asia Minor, that was known in antiquity as Caria. Hence, mention of the city in an archaeological context usually appears as "Aphrodisias in Caria", in order to distinguish it from a few other cities with a similar name.

There can be no doubt, however, that Carian Aphrodisias was the most famous among these. The first-century BC geographer, Strabo, is the only ancient author who included it among the cities of the neighbouring province of Phrygia. Writing much later, in the sixth century, the grammarian and encyclopaedist Stephanus of Byzantium listed it among the border towns between Lydia and Caria. Ancient geographical limits were not rigidly fixed: so one may conclude from the written sources that, although technically in Caria, Aphrodisias lay close to the confines of Lydia (to the north-west) and Phrygia (to the north-east).

Stephanus briefly and unwittingly provides an interesting insight into its remote past and its tradition as a city. He mentions Aphrodisias under the entry for the obsolete name Ninoë, observing that it was "founded by the Pelasgian Leleges, then called Lelegonopolis, subsequently Megalè Polis (the Great City) then, after Ninos, Ninoë." The reference to the Pelasgians and Leleges, two pre-Greek 'aboriginal' Aegean peoples or tribes variously located in Greece or Asia Minor, is hardly useful, except for implying great, or 'prehistoric' antiquity. The mention of Ninos, on the other hand, though equally vague, is more thought-provoking. According to Greek tradition, Ninos was the son of Belos, or Bel, a divine

From a restored relief originally in the Sebasteion, built in his divine memory and in honour of his descendants, the emperor Augustus once more surveys his favoured city, as it is slowly resurrected.

25

Ninos, the mythical founder of Ninoë, later called Aphrodisias, is shown on a balustrade relief panel in Roman imperial garb, performing a sacrifice by an altar on which an eagle stands with wings spread out. He is identified by an inscription above his head, shown partly in detail *opposite*. However, his military companion (also performing a sacrifice), the three-branched tree trunk in front of him, and the context of the action of Ninos, cannot be interpreted as they all undoubtedly pertained to the foundation legends of the city, of which we have no knowledge.

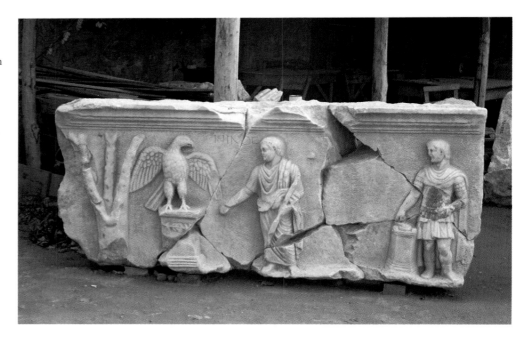

equivalent of the Greek god Kronos. He was the mythical founder of the Assyro-Babylonian empire and of the city of Nineveh, and, eventually, husband to Semiramis. He is purported to have conquered most of western Asia as far as the Aegean. It is more than likely that the details reported so briefly by Stephanus echoed much earlier foundation legends that had in turn grown from some vague traditions in the late Hellenistic period (the second to the first centuries BC) which surrounded cities like Aphrodisias, to provide them with a more heroic or glorious past.

Interestingly, archaeological evidence has verified the accuracy of some of Stephanus' assertions. In 1977, a large basilica was partly excavated off the south-western corner of the agora of Aphrodisias. Relief panels decorating the balustrade of an upper storey portrayed figures which were identified with inscriptions: among these were Ninos and Semiramis. On stylistic and archaeological grounds, the reliefs can be dated to the second half of the third century BC. They clearly imply that the tradition of a connection with Ninos was well established by that time and was not a misinterpretation on the part of Stephanus.

Although Stephanus the encyclopaedist was correct about the association with Ninos, in his role as grammarian he was unable to explain the etymological implications of the names Ninos and Ninoë. Archaeological deduction suggests a connection with Nin or Nanai, the Akkadian appellation for Ishtar (also known as Astarte), the Mesopotamian goddess of love and war. The Carian site was associated with the Greek Aphrodite in the late Hellenistic period, probably at the same time as a foundation legend was elaborated. Consequently the name Aphrodisias, which was used when Aphrodite was worshipped here, may be regarded as the Hellenistic equivalent of Ninoë.

There was a turning point in the history of Aphrodisias at this time, probably connected with the full establishment of Roman power in western Asia in the late Hellenistic period. Before this, Aphrodisias had not actually been a city in the full sense of the word. It had been a sacred or temple site, featuring a sanctuary and its associated buildings, along with a reasonably extensive population tending to the needs of the cult as well as to the fields and to the requirements of other properties around.

The cult itself must have extended back to great antiquity, like many others in Asia Minor, perhaps even to prehistoric times. A number of small 'idols' found in the excavations of the prehistoric mounds might well be the first manifestations of the goddess who was eventually to become identified with Aphrodite. It is reasonable to assume that at this early stage the personality of this goddess was dictated by the essentially agricultural activities of the inhabitants and the great fertility of the soil of the area. In other words, she was a local version of the numerous 'mother nature' or fertility divinities

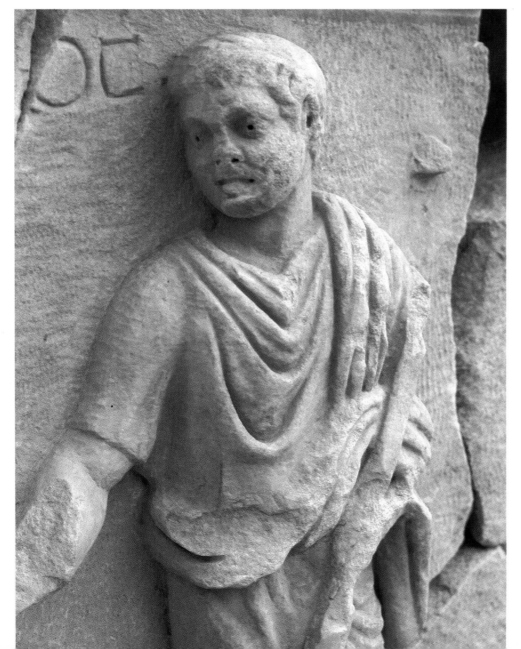

Detail of Ninos, from the balustrade relief (*opposite*). This relief was part of the decoration added to the large basilica, or administrative centre, which stood by the southern part of the Portico of Tiberius of the Agora. It is dated to the second half of the third century AD, when Aphrodisias became for a while the capital of a joint province of Caria-Phrygia.

Small marble and other stone 'idols' – possibly fertility figures – from the Bronze Age, have been found in prehistoric excavations at Aphrodisias.

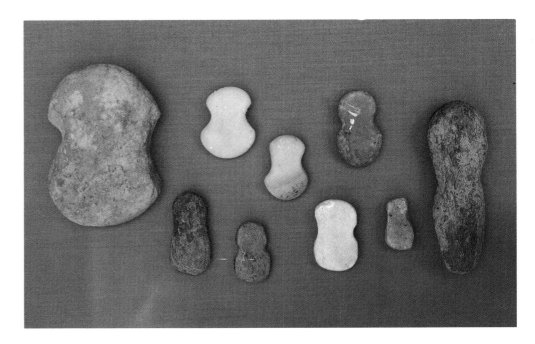

that prevailed in Anatolia as well as in other parts of western Asia from Neolithic times onward.

Several of the better known Anatolian manifestations of this fertility goddess came to assume the name of Cybele or Artemis — the latter most notably at Ephesus and Magnesia-on-the-Maeander. It is possible, however, that influences from the east and Mesopotamia were eventually grafted on to the local Carian traditions of her cult. These influences may have brought with them names such as Nina, Nin, Nana or Enana. As we have seen, her equation with Aphrodite — who was herself not a fully Greek goddess but one with eastern affiliations — appears to have occurred relatively late, in the second or first century BC.

The establishment of Roman rule in Asia Minor at that time may well have encouraged the association of the sanctuary with Aphrodite, and the concomitant change of the growing city's name to Aphrodisias. These would have been shrewd political moves by the priests or elders of the city, as the Romans claimed descent from the Trojan prince Aeneas, who was a son of the goddess Venus, the Roman goddess equated with the Greek Aphrodite. Another motive for changing the city's name may simply have been the growing reputation in the Roman world of the Aphrodisian sanctuary: its renown spread far beyond the frontiers of Caria and western Asia Minor. According to Appian, the second century AD Roman historian, the oracle of Apollo at Delphi advised the Roman dictator Sulla to make offerings to his favourite divinity Aphrodite at her Carian shrine in order to obtain good fortune and power. Sulla is reported to have donated a golden crown and a double axe in 81 BC. The latter was undoubtedly a suitable gift for the goddess, not only as a weapon symbolising war and power, but also as a frequently used Carian emblem.

The name of Aphrodisias appears in the late second to early first century BC on several modest bronze and silver coins. However, it is regularly accompanied on these by the name of Plarasa, a neighbouring town, with which the coins were jointly issued. Plarasa may have been located near the present village of Bingeç about fourteen kilometres south-west of Aphrodisias-Geyre and was associated with the city of Aphrodite in a 'sympolity', or close political or religious union. Of the two, Plarasa may have boasted a more ancient background: its name usually precedes that of Aphrodisia on coins and in other references. Under the Roman empire, however, Plarasa disappears from all documents. It seems likely that the rich sanctuary site of Aphrodisias, located in the fertile but unprotected plain, was enabled to supersede or absorb Plarasa after Roman rule brought peace to the area.

Many inscribed documents — some linking Aphrodisias and Plarasa — were discovered in 1969 carved on the northern, so-called 'Archive', wall of the stage building of the Aphrodisias Theatre. These include a series of letters emanating from emperors, from the first to the third centuries AD. Several of the inscriptions offer important information not only concerning Aphrodisias' history, but also about aspects of Roman policy in Asia Minor. They also provide interesting insights into the period following Julius Caesar's assassination in 44 BC and the subsequent rule of the Second Triumvirate composed of Mark Antony, Octavian and Lepidus who controlled the Roman world from 43-31 BC. These inscriptions constitute a remarkable record of Aphrodisias' relationship with Rome. One of the early inscriptions mentions a gold statue of Eros dedicated by Julius Caesar to Aphrodite, which accentuates our impression of the reputation of the Carian goddess abroad. Caesar's family, the *gens* Julia, claimed direct descent from Venus; the dedication therefore suggests that the Aphrodisians had already begun to establish ties with Caesar and the Julian family via their goddess before the dictator's assassination.

After Caesar's murder, Brutus and Cassius, his assassins, withdrew from Italy to Asia Minor. While there is no complete evidence as to what happened at Aphrodisias, the city's territory appears to have been invaded, which suggests that the Aphrodisians remained loyal to Caesar's cause. Brutus and Cassius were defeated at Pharsalus in 42 BC. In 40 BC, however, one of their supporters, Q. Labienus, invaded western Asia Minor, with support from the eastern empire of the Parthians. The documents on the Archive Wall make it clear that the city was attacked, and that both the sanctuary and private property were plundered before Labienus was defeated by Antony in 39 BC.

Although Aphrodisias lay in the sphere of influence ceded to Antony, later inscriptions found, in part, on the Archive Wall of the Theatre reveal that Octavian, Caesar's great-nephew and heir, was able to resume the personal and political ties established by Caesar

29

with the citizens of Aphrodisias and their goddess. An Aphrodisian by the name of Zoilos, who was perhaps inherited as a slave from the household of Caesar and later freed by Octavian, played a major role in keeping the city loyal to the cause of Caesar's family. He was also instrumental in obtaining a grant of special status to his native city. Indeed, in 39 BC, after the departure of Labienus' army, Aphrodisias was the recipient of special privileges via a triumviral decree, a senatorial decree (*senatus consultum*), a treaty and a law. These documents, all inscribed on the Archive Wall, granted the city freedom, a non-taxable status and increased asylum rights of inviolability in Aphrodite's sanctuary. The influence wielded by Octavian in these decisions was unquestionably strong. In one inscribed document, a letter, Octavian referred warmly to Zoilos as a close and "esteemed friend" and to Aphrodisias as the "one city from all of Asia" (meaning the Roman province bearing that name in western Asia Minor) that he selected as his own. These feelings did not change when Octavian became Emperor Augustus in 27 BC and continued under his successors.

A Julio-Claudian prince from a relief from the Sebasteion , in the process of being crowned with a wreath.

From the late first century BC Aphrodisias the city enjoyed a long period of prosperity, as well as of remarkable cultural and artistic renown. Its sculptors, skilfully using the excellent marble sources in

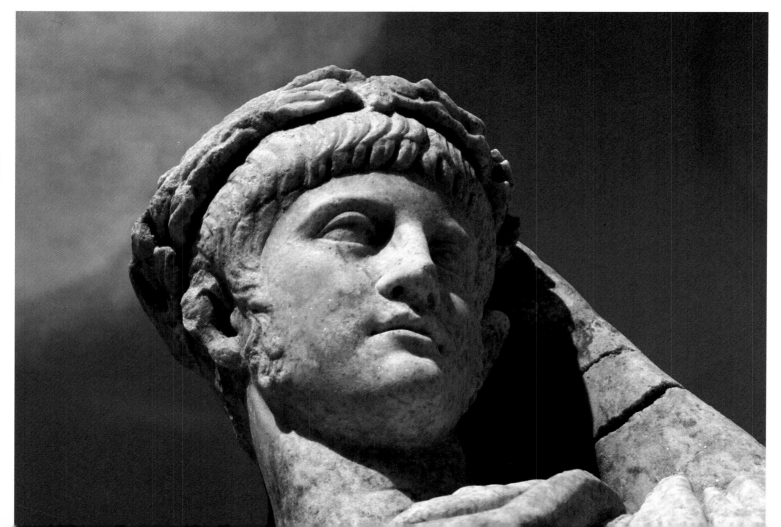

quarries situated to the east of the city, began to refine their talents and rapidly gained prominence at home and abroad, especially in Rome and elsewhere in Italy, as creative artists and fine craftsmen of marble. Elaborate monuments were also erected in Aphrodisias itself from the late first century BC onward, partly to restore earlier depredations or to complete interrupted building programmes, and partly to pay distinctive honour to Rome and its emperors.

The sanctuary of Aphrodite attracted increasing numbers of pilgrims and visitors from far and wide. Thus the city became not only an important religious and artistic centre, but also a centre for literary, scientific and other intellectual endeavours. In the first centuries AD, Aphrodisias' talented sons included Xenocrates, who wrote treatises on medicine, and Chariton, one of the earliest writers of ancient romances and novels. His *Chaereas and Callirhoe*, is considered among the better specimens of the ancient romantic literary genre.

A series of letters from emperors of the second and third centuries AD (ranging from Trajan to Gordian III and Decius), most of which were inscribed on the Archive Wall of the Theatre, testify to the continuing privileged status of Aphrodisias and the maintenance of a close relationship with the central authority in Rome. Modern archaeological discoveries in Rome and elsewhere around the Mediterranean indicate that during the second century AD the reputation of the Carian sculptors reached new heights. Oratory and phil-

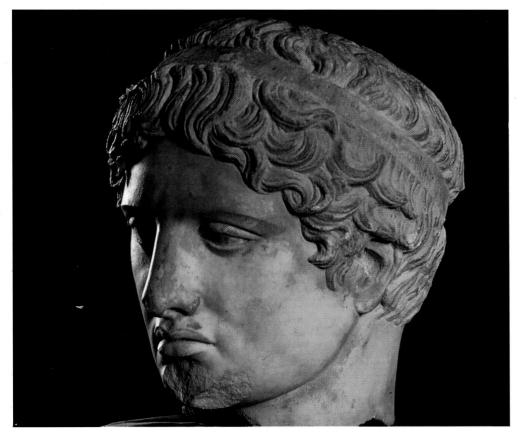

The head of a life-size statue of an athlete, inspired by the so-called Diskophoros figure created by the famous fifth-century BC sculptor Polykleitos, still bears traces of colour. It is easy to forget that ancient marble statuary was subtly coloured, although flesh parts were usually left in the original colour of the stone.

31

osophy also flourished at Aphrodisias, and at the close of the second century, the Aphrodisian Alexander — still regarded today as being one of the most able commentators on Aristotle's work — lectured at Athens on the master's philosophy.

In contrast, the third century was a difficult period for Aphrodisias. There were drastic changes in the administration of the empire and, as a result, in the status of many cities and regions. The autonomy enjoyed until then by Aphrodisias, and by other privileged cities, ceased. Epigraphic documents found in excavations in recent years suggest gradual modifications of its special position. They reveal that a new combined province of Caria and Phrygia was apparently created in the 250s. Although a free city and prior to that date reckoned as part of the province of Asia, Aphrodisias probably acted as the administrative centre of the new unit. Subsequently, under Diocletian (284–305), it became the capital, or metropolis, of a smaller province of Caria.

At first glance, the location of Aphrodisias may appear to be remote from the main centres of communication in the Mediterranean basin in classical times. In local terms (*see inset*), Aphrodisias was situated on a fertile high plateau, well-watered by the springs descending from the Baba Dağ range and the various streams that formed from them and ultimately flowed into the Maeander. The inhabitants of the higher and more remote plateau of nearby Tabae (modern Tavas), where the towns of Heraclaea and Apollonia were located, were clearly inclined to communicate more readily with Aphrodisias and the Maeander valley beyond, than with other centres to the north, east and south. The shrine at Aphrodisias and the later city maintained easy contact with larger commercial centres or ports. This was particularly so in Imperial times. The export of Aphrodisian marble and partly finished sculpture was probably undertaken by ox-cart or occasionally by river transport down the Maeander to the coast, from where it was shipped to Rome and other parts of the Mediterranean.

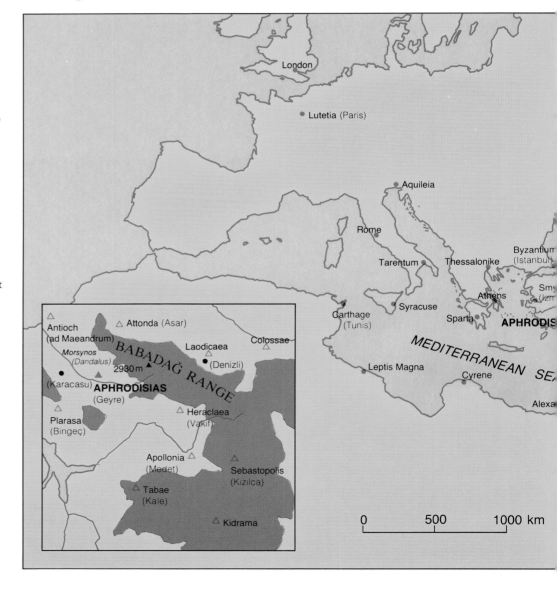

With the Empire's adoption of Christianity in the fourth century, the city's administrative position favoured the establishment of an archbishopric. The earliest known name of an Aphrodisian bishop is that of Ammonius, who participated in the Council of Nicaea in 325. Two early Christian martyrs, apparently put to death under Diocletian, were also ascribed to the city. Yet the cult of the fertility goddess had played an essential role in the life and history of the city for well over 1,000 years, and such measures could not immediately eradicate the deeply-rooted pagan tradition.

In the course of the fifth and sixth centuries several bishops of the city, with the support of their fellow citizens, became deeply involved in the theological disputes and heresies concerning the nature of Christ that perturbed the period. The monophysites, who believed that the divine and human elements in Christ were inseparable, but that his divinity was of overriding importance, proved to be particularly active at Aphrodisias. In 518, Euphemius, even

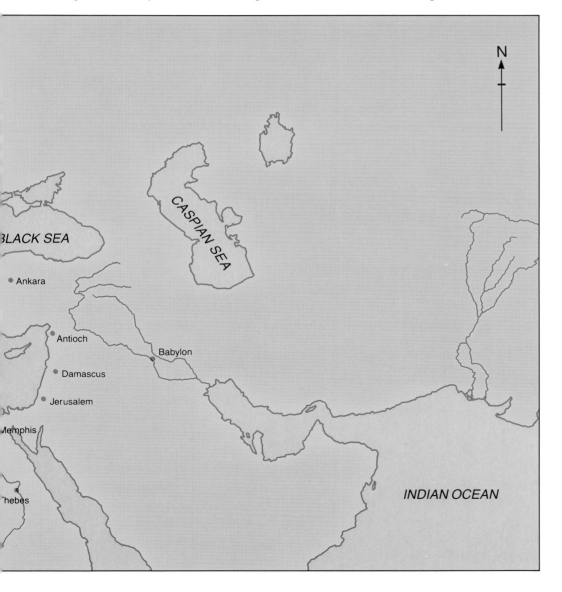

though he was bishop of the city, was expelled for his heretical monophysite activities. At the same time, paganism and pagan teaching was still vigorous at the city, and there are references to pagan sacrifice that can be dated as late as 484.

During this period, at least one distinguished pagan philosopher, the Alexandrian Asklepiodotos, chose to work and teach at Aphrodisias. There is considerable evidence that both pagans and Christians made generous benefactions to the city. Another benefactor was Emperor Justinian. Evidence shows that in, or shortly after, 529, the people of Aphrodisias petitioned him to protect the interest payments which they received from these endowments. This he did, and the substantial sum of money that was saved as a result went to meet civic costs such as the heating of the baths.

It was under Justinian that a concentrated attempt was made to eradicate paganism in western Asia Minor; it was perhaps at this time that the words 'Aphrodisias' and 'Aphrodisian' were systematically erased on most local inscriptions. Attempts were also made in the sixth, or certainly the seventh, century to impose the name 'Stavropolis' (or 'City of the Cross') in place of 'Aphrodisias'. Although Stavropolis occasionally occurs in several Byzantine contexts after the seventh century, the city gradually came to be referred to simply as 'Caria', probably because it continued to be the chief urban centre in the area. The name of the Turkish village of Geyre stems from that Byzantine use of Caria.

Information concerning Aphrodisias-Caria between the fourth and eleventh centuries is sketchy, and comes mostly from epigraphic sources. The archaeological evidence is in the process of being studied and evaluated.

In the mid-fourth century, the city, which does not appear to have had any specific earlier fortifications, was endowed with ambitious perimeter walls, about three and a half kilometers in circumference, which enclosed the city's major portion in a roughly circular or polygonal fashion.

In the late 350s the city was apparently devastated by one or more earthquakes that caused the collapse of many of its major monuments. The extent of the damage was revealed in the course of our excavations, which have also produced evidence suggesting that the cataclysm created havoc with the ground water table of the whole site and particularly affected the canalizations of the city, resulting in serious flooding of the lower lying areas. Some of the buildings were restored in the fifth century, but the remnants of others were re-used freely in the restoration of the fortification walls. Various attempts were also made to remedy the causes of the flooding, but usually only with limited success. Later earthquakes may have further exacerbated the problem, which is still evident today in some excavated areas particularly at the edge of the Agora.

Like many other cities of the late Roman Empire and of the early Byzantine Empire — which succeeded Rome in the eastern Mediterranean — Aphrodisias managed at first to hold its own and maintained its importance until the seventh century. But there was a steady diminution over this period in the vitality of the ancient cities which had been the centres of political and cultural life in the area for at least 1,000 years. Aphrodisias was no exception to this general trend.

In the seventh century, the threat of Persian invasion caused serious concern. Simultaneously, another catastrophic earthquake, which probably took place in the reign of Heraclius (610-641), appears to have sapped whatever was left of the city's civic energy. Many of the monuments damaged by this second disaster could not be repaired and were left in ruins. Only essential restoration was attempted. The high conical mound into which the ancient theatre had been built, was surrounded by walls and transformed into a citadel, where the dwindling population could take refuge in times of danger. This hillock — mistakenly called the 'Acropolis' by previous archaeologists because of its prominent position — would have acted as an excellent look-out point since the long perimeter of the old fourth century fortification system could not be adequately manned for this purpose.

The names of some of the later bishops of Aphrodisias can be gleaned from various patriarchal documents. The name of the see of Aphrodisias still occurs as late as the fourteenth century, when it is mentioned as being in considerable difficulty; and it appears that the titular bishop was no longer resident.

Between the eleventh and thirteenth centuries, the appearance and eventual establishment of the Seljuk Turks in Anatolia and its western confines followed by raids by Turkoman horsemen, doomed many urban centres of the interior valleys. Contemporary Byzantine sources such as Nicetas Choniates and George Pachymeres, from the twelfth or thirteenth century, testify to at least four captures of 'Caria' by the Turks, presumably with brief intervening periods of recovery.

After the thirteenth century, and the voluntary resettlement of many of its remaining inhabitants elsewhere by the Turks, the site of Aphrodisias (alias Caria) was virtually abandoned. The area became part of the *beylik* (principality) of Aydin (ancient Tralles) and, according to some sources, it was also part of the *beylik* of Menteşe for a while. Eventually the fertility of the area and its abundant water supply attracted settlers to the ruined site of the city. A Turkish village named Geyre grew among the ruins of the once splendid monuments. There is little clear evidence concerning earlier periods of Geyre, but it is mentioned from the seventeenth century onward by travellers to this area. The inhabitants they met there may even have been descendants of earlier Aphrodisians.

35

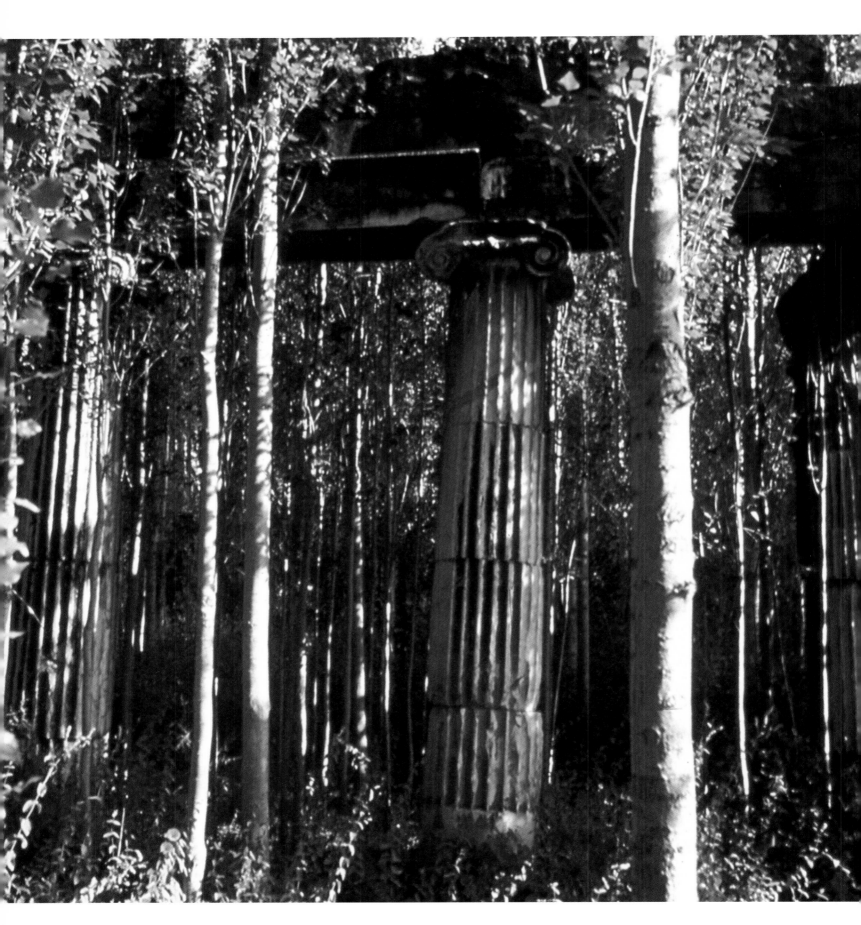

CHAPTER THREE

Early Reports and Excavations

When European travellers began to explore the antiquities of western Anatolia, principally from the eighteenth century, the ancient city of Aphrodisias was half-forgotten. Unlike some other ancient sites, however, it was never quite 'lost'. Despite countless disasters and the many changes of name given to the city in the course of its decline, the location of its site at the Turkish village of Geyre was never in doubt.

Aphrodisias was not always indicated on maps purporting to give an accurate geographical view of classical Asia Minor, however, and it may be partly for this reason that some travellers failed to mention the site. Some, although by no means all, were undoubtedly daunted by the difficulty of access to the area. The deterioration of the Roman road connecting Aphrodisias to the Maeander valley in Byzantine times, and the subsequent growth of the town of Karacasu during the Ottoman period, had further isolated the former city and shrine of Aphrodite.

Despite one or two earlier reports and illustrated accounts, most that feature Aphrodisias in some detail belong to the late eighteenth, and especially the nineteenth, centuries. Several of these include maps, plans, drawings or engravings, copies of texts of inscriptions and more or less accurate descriptions of the visible remains. One of the two most extensive accounts is to be found in Volume III (1840) of the *Antiquities of Ionia*. This series of five volumes, published between 1769 and 1915, describes the results of expeditions by English architects and draughtsmen — notably Sir William Gell and Mr John Peter Gandy, who later changed his name to Deering — to Asia Minor and Greece, organized by the Society of Dilettanti from the late eighteenth century on. Equally full, although less reliable, is Charles Texier's *Description de l'Asie Mineure*, Volume III (1849). Texier described, with a number of mistakes and a fair amount of imagination, the monuments of Asia Minor, including those of Aphrodisias which he saw during a visit in 1835. Despite their inevitable shortcomings, inaccuracies and misinterpretations, these early reports are always most useful for giving an idea of the

The uniquely romantic character of Aphrodisias is epitomized by the extraordinarily happy blend of its remains and their natural setting, as these stately columns of the Agora exemplify, still standing surrounded by groves of poplar trees.

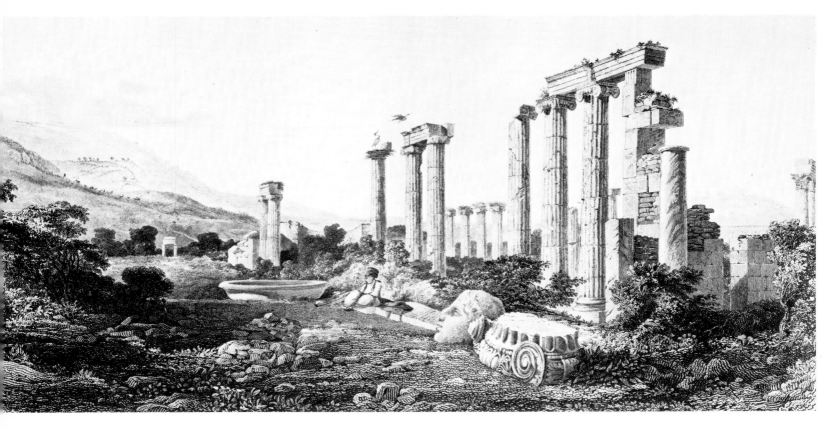

The Temple of Aphrodite, as portrayed in an engraving from *The Antiquities of Ionia* (1840).

Work in progress at the Baths of Hadrian during Gaudin's excavations in 1904.

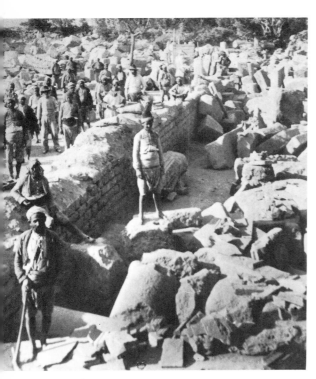

remains of the ancient city as they appeared to the visitor two centuries or so ago.

If the remote location and difficulty of access were not insurmountable obstacles to eighteenth- and nineteenth-century travellers, they presented more serious problems for a systematic investigation and excavation. In 1892, Osman Hamdi Bey, then Director General of the Imperial Museum in Constantinople, paid a visit to Aphrodisias and was impressed. He resolved to launch an excavation there and obtained a permit from the Ottoman authorities to begin work. Unfortunately, practical and financial considerations prevented Hamdi Bey from carrying out his plans. The mission to explore Aphrodisias was then entrusted by him in 1904 to a French engineer resident in Smyrna, named Paul Gaudin, who was also a collector of antiquities and devotee of archaeology. At the time, Gaudin was Director of the Smyrna-Kassaba railroad and, therefore, had at his disposal financial means and equipment not available to Hamdi Bey.

The first campaign lasted for about six weeks in the summer of 1904. Gaudin acted as field director with a staff composed of a surveyor, some supervisory personnel, a photographer and a representative of the Imperial Museum. The number of workmen and foremen employed reached almost a hundred. A general reconnaissance of the site and a plan were completed first. Although the

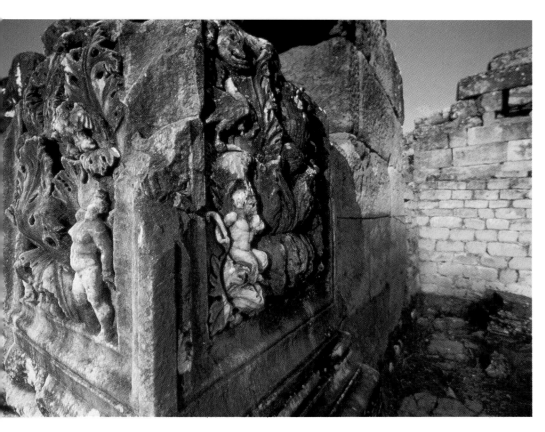

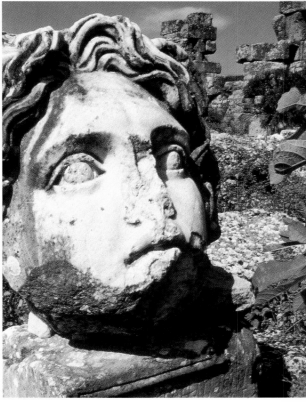

The lower portion of a pillar, decorated in the 'peopled scrolls' manner, remains *in situ* in the front court of the Baths of Hadrian (*above left*).

A fragmentary colossal head (*above*), possibly of Perseus, of the type found by Gaudin and left at the site.

active digging season proved to be relatively short and the work exploratory, several soundings and large-scale excavations were undertaken in at least thirty-eight areas. The main points on which investigations concentrated included the Temple of Aphrodite, the late Roman-Byzantine fortification system, parts of the city's vast necropolis, a so-called gymnasium and a vast complex of ruins, which was first thought to be a basilica, but later turned out to be a large bathing establishment dedicated to the emperor Hadrian (hence its name: Baths of Hadrian). A huge amount of architectural decoration and sculptural finds were collected from these excavations, while over two hundred inscriptions were recorded, including many official documents. Most of these dated to the first five centuries of the Christian era. The building of a roadway was commenced between Geyre and Kızılca Bölük fifty kilometres to the south-east, for the eventual transport of equipment and antiquities.

Despite a widespread lack of interest in Graeco-Roman sites early in this century, the results of Gaudin's first campaign were so impressive that they attracted the attention of established French archaeologists and scholars. In consequence, a second campaign was planned for 1905, with financial assistance from French official sources and the appointment of two scientific collaborators to Gaudin. One of these was Gustav Mendel, of the University of Bordeaux. The 1905 season started in late August and again focused on the continuation of work in the Baths of Hadrian and in the Temple of Aphrodite.

This fragment of the 'peopled scrolls' pilaster (*below*) discovered at the Baths of Hadrian during Gaudin's excavation in 1904, was subsequently transported, along with other architectural and sculptural finds, to the then Imperial Museum at Constantinople, today the Archaeological Museums in Istanbul.

The Baths of Hadrian (*below right*) betrayed just such an abandoned but still profoundly compelling appearance to us when we first visited Aphrodisias in 1959. Contrary to her reputation, Medusa's face had an almost imploring look, which was particularly moving, and contrasted dramatically with the usual, more formidable, aspect, illustrated opposite.

Work had barely begun, however, when Gaudin was suddenly appointed to the Directorate of the Hejaz railroad by order of the Sultan Abdul Hamid II and had to depart for Syria and Arabia, leaving Mendel in charge. It is fairly safe to assume that this sudden appointment was in great part due to behind-the-scenes intrigues, undoubtedly fanned by hostility felt towards Gaudin, who was considered an amateur and an outsider by some members of the French School in Athens. Nevertheless, Gaudin clearly intended to resume his leadership of the excavations in the course of his summer holidays. Unfortunately, this plan was thwarted by a variety of circumstances, including the worsening international political situation as well as continued animosity towards him from French scholarly circles.

Not surprisingly, in 1913 the French School in Athens applied to the new Director General of the Imperial Museum in Constantinople, Halil Edhem Bey (Hamdi Bey had died in the interim) for

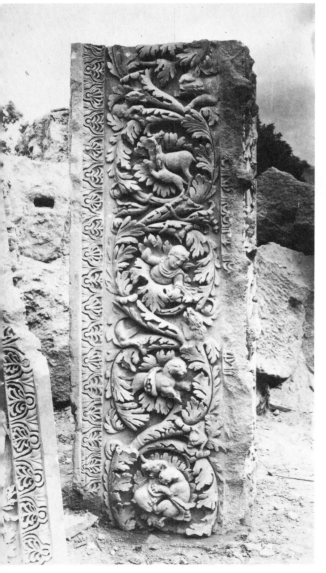

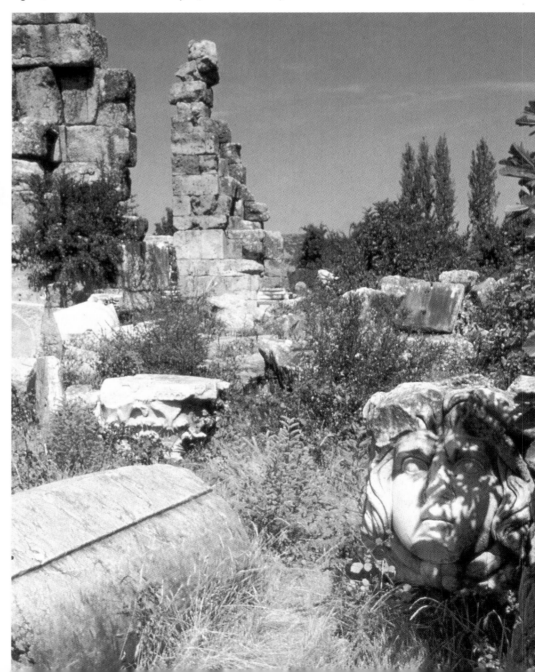

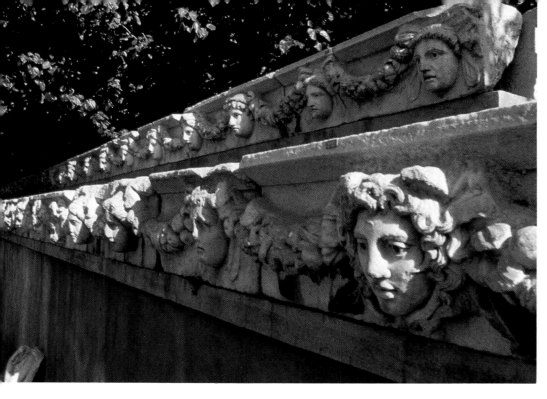

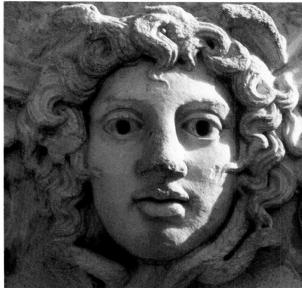

permission to resume the Aphrodisias excavations. The new leader was to be one of the School's members, André Boulanger. Although the request was favourably received, inexplicable delays prevented a full-scale campaign. Boulanger's work was limited to activities near the Baths of Hadrian in the autumn of that year. The following year, the outbreak of The First World War brought an end to any hope of work at Aphrodisias in the immediate future.

In fact, excavations were not to be resumed for another twenty-four years. In 1937, an Italian mission headed by Giulio Jacopi was granted permission by the Turkish authorities to start its own investigations. These were also affected by a series of problems, including the growing tensions in the international political scene, and were consequently short-lived. Nevertheless, over a period of several weeks in the autumn, Jacopi and his collaborators managed to make good progress. Their excavations centred in the Agora area of the city and revealed part of one of its two Ionic porticoes dedicated to the emperor Tiberius. Their most stunning discovery was the frieze of the portico which featured an amazingly well-preserved array of handsome masks joined by garlands. The results of the Italian excavations were published just before the outbreak of the Second World War in 1939.

Unfortunately, Gaudin's earlier activities were not so well served: only brief reports, and some more detailed accounts of a number of inscriptions, were published in scholarly journals. The inadequacy of the record may be partly explained by the dispersal after the First World War of much of the uncovered material and its documentation. Most of the major and well-preserved statuary and architectural fragments were transported in 1905 and 1906 to the then Imperial Museum in Constantinople (now the Archaeological Museums in Istanbul). These included an impressive series of full-length portrait statues, splendidly decorated pilasters ('peopled

A less pathetic Medusa *(above)* decorated the typically Aphrodisian frieze of garlanded masks and faces *(above left)* that topped the Ionic Portico of Tiberius of the Agora. The sculptural quality of most of these heads is remarkable, as the bearded face *(below)* shows. Many series of blocks from this frieze (now in the Archaeological Museum at Basmane, in Izmir) were unearthed in 1937 by G. Jacopi.

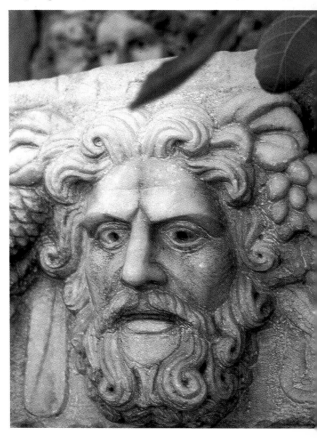

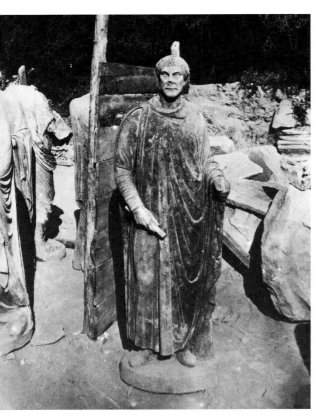

Photographed on its discovery by Gaudin in 1904, this full portrait statue represented a high official wearing the long *chlamys* fashionable in the fifth century AD.

scrolls') with handsome lintels and capitals, colossal console heads and other sculpture and relief fragments, most of which came from the Baths of Hadrian.

Following Jacopi's excavations of 1937, the most striking and well-preserved specimens of the mask-and-garlands frieze of the Portico of Tiberius were removed from Geyre to the Archaeological Museum in Izmir (at Basmane), along with several items left over from Gaudin's expedition of 1904-1905. These are still there but they are rather difficult to get to and are poorly displayed. Prospects for their eventual transfer and exhibition in the recently completed Izmir Archaeological Museum appear promising, although the best solution would be to return them to Aphrodisias and restore them over the re-erected columns of the portico.

Shortly after our work began at Aphrodisias in 1961, we were lucky enough to make contact with Monsieur Albert Gaudin, in Versailles, and the late Professor Antoine Gaudin, of the Massachusetts Institute of Technology, both sons of the first excavator of the site. They generously gave us access to a series of documents, including photographs from their father's files, as well as actual antiquities. This documentation revealed much intriguing new information, as did our subsequent consultation of the archives and correspondence dossiers of the Archaeological Museums in Istanbul. In order to solve the riddle of the many items that were missing, we decided to embark on some detective work.

From the correspondence between Hamdi Bey and Paul Gaudin, it was possible to surmise that arrangements had been made between them to allow some of the finds to be made over to Gaudin after the 1904 campaign, in compensation, as it were, for his financing the excavations. Gaudin, at any rate, submitted a list of his desiderata. Nevertheless, his request, which was supported by a petition filed by Hamdi Bey in 1905, did not result in positive official action, and in the following year the removal of antiquities from the country was specifically prohibited by a new Turkish law.

It furthermore appears that important pieces of sculpture had been illegally exported without notification to Hamdi Bey after the 1904 campaign, and more followed even after the promulgation of the 1906 law. The presence of a bearded head in the collections of the Musée du Cinquantenaire in Brussels, and an old fisherman's torso in the Altes Museum in Berlin can only lead to such troubling conclusions, since both pieces are well-represented among Gaudin's photographic records. Furthermore, following Gaudin's death in 1922, Madame Veuve Gaudin continued to write to the Directorate of the Archaeological Museums and lay claim to the pieces requested by her husband. Halil Edhem Bey, the Director General, retorted

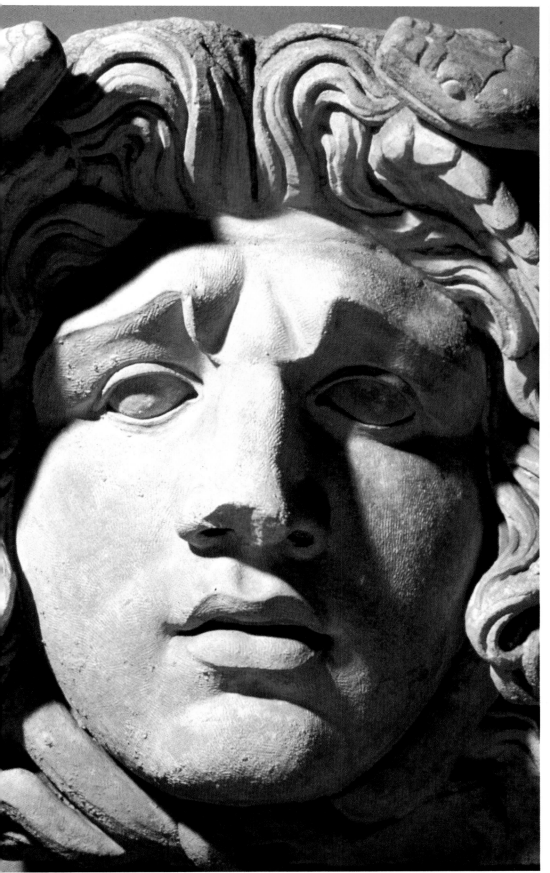

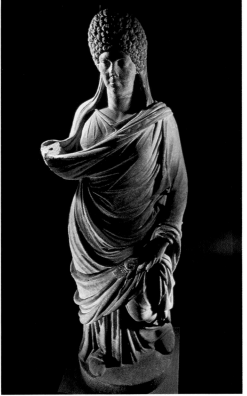

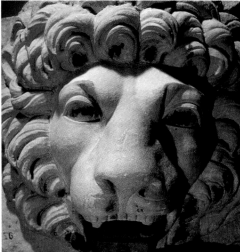

Found near the Baths of Hadrian like the figure opposite, this elegant lady portrayed a well-to-do matron of the early second century AD.

The Medusa head and the lion, left and above, formed part of a series of colossal consoles that decorated the forecourt of the Baths of Hadrian. All date from the second century AD, and are now in Istanbul.

that complaints had been voiced about the Gaudins' surreptitious shipment of eight crates out of Smyrna to France.

Between 1922 and 1931, Madame Gaudin was forced by circumstances to sell part of her collection of antiquities, both privately and at public auction, and undoubtedly items found at Aphrodisias were included. Unfortunately, the descriptions of the pieces offered for sale in the catalogues of the Hôtel Drouot, the Paris auction house, are too brief to enable them to be matched with photographs of unidentified items of sculpture, or with the lists kept by Madame Gaudin. Nevertheless, an attractive under-lifesize figure of a Negro, carved in black marble and listed as coming from Aphrodisias, was not sold and remains in the possession of Monsieur and Madame Albert Gaudin in Versailles. Two other items, traceable through photographs, but purchased by dealers — who subsequently sold them respectively to the Nycarlsberg Glyptotek in Copenhagen and the Boston Museum of Fine Arts — were one female head (Faustina the Younger or Lucilla) and one male head of the fifth century.

Through an extraordinary set of circumstances a fragment, once in the Gaudin collection at Versailles, featuring the upper left eye, cheek and forehead of a bearded male portrait of the fifth century, was able to be joined to the rest of its head in 1984, when the latter was discovered in clearing operations in the area excavated by Gaudin in 1904. Several additional handsome portrait heads, male torsos and other fragments are known only through faded photographs, and remain unaccounted for.

Both the fifth-century bearded portrait head (now in Brussels) and the old fisherman's torso (in Berlin) shown here in original Gaudin photographs, were unfortunately removed from Aphrodisias following their discovery in 1904.

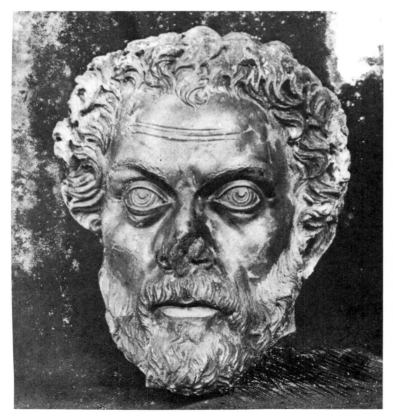

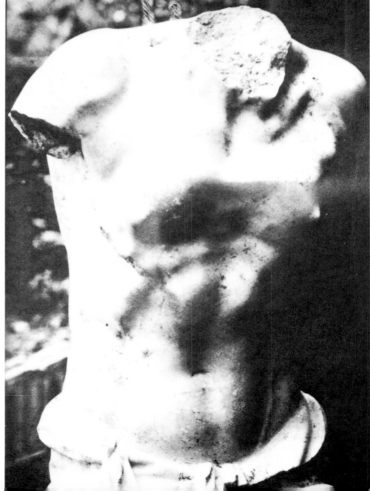

44

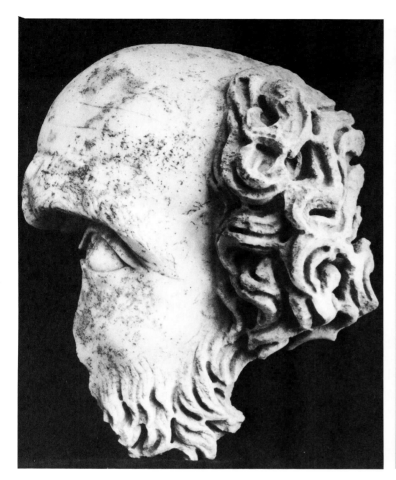

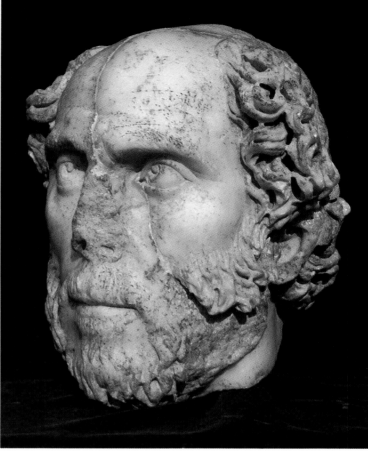

Documents located by Monsieur Albert Gaudin, including letters and a plan of a garden once belonging to a relative of his family in Bornova, near Izmir, indicate that a number of pieces of sculpture that apparently could not be shipped out of Turkey were buried there in an attempt to thwart confiscation by Turkish authorities in 1926. The accuracy of this information was verified thanks to the identification of a fragmentary sarcophagus panel, shown in a Gaudin photograph and now in the Izmir Archaeological Museum (at Basmane). The register of the Museum did not record the Aphrodisian origin of the panel, but reported that it was unearthed, following a denunciation, in a property in Bornova! Several additional fragments whose burial locations are marked on the plan of the garden are still missing, which suggests that excavations relating to Aphrodisias should perhaps also be conducted at Bornova.

The 'detective' work described above illustrates well the problems confronting all archaeologists in their search for, and research of, material excavated in earlier days. It also gives an indication of the extraordinary quantity of sculptural finds made at Aphrodisias since the early years of this century. Regrettably, it has also shown that some of the pioneering excavators cared less than we do today about the need to retain unearthed treasures in their original and proper context.

This fragment of a fifth-century portrait head (*above left*), was apparently taken to France by Gaudin, after its discovery in 1904. It remained in the possession of Gaudin's family until the author was permitted to return it to Aphrodisias. The remainder of the head, with which the fragment can be seen united (*above right*) was not discovered until 1984, however, eighty years after the original smaller piece had been lifted from the ground.

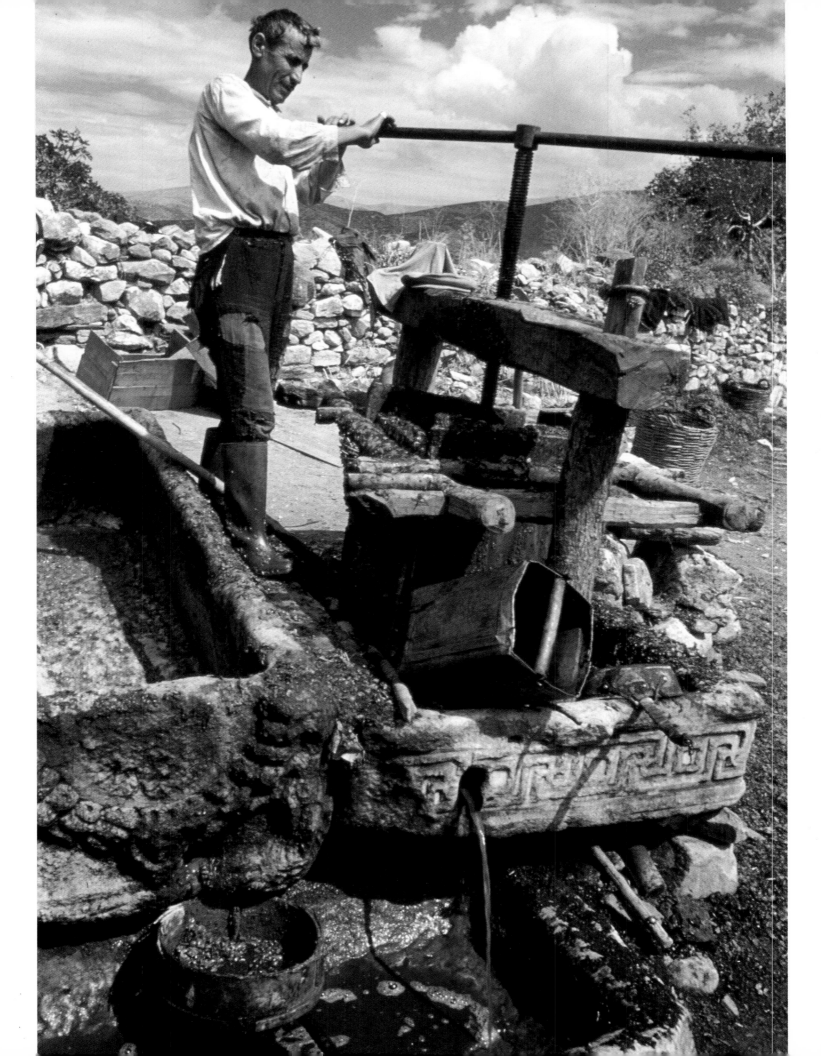

CHAPTER FOUR

Recent Discoveries

Excavations today are not undertaken for the sake of collecting works of art and ancient artefacts, nor simply for the thrill of digging or treasure-hunting, as they were all too often in the past. Modern archaeologists are motivated by questions of scholarly interest, and archaeological expeditions are mounted in order to further knowledge about a culture, a site, an important geographical area, or a particular period of history or prehistory. Furthermore most archaeologists are aware of the need to protect or salvage sites threatened by looters or the encroachments of modern life. An excavation in the late twentieth century resembles in many ways a laboratory in which the views and the theories of historians and other scholars can be tested against the physical evidence unearthed by the archaeologists.

In archaeology, as in other fields, there are unfortunately today certain favoured trends: 'fashionable' geographical areas, historic or prehistoric periods, and occasionally excessive reliance on sophisticated scientific techniques. Although science undoubtedly facilitates the work of the archaeologist, it must not be forgotten that archaeology is a humanistic enterprise which should not be dominated by complicated charts, statistics, and laboratory tests intelligible only to specialists. Alas, the archaeologist soon becomes aware that trend and fashion also have effect on the financing of many projects. It is fortunate, however, that not all such trends are invidious or ephemeral.

One fortunate tendency is the now widely shared belief that objects and artefacts must be studied and maintained within their context at or near the site where they were found. This sentiment has led to the formulation of the 1970 UNESCO Convention concerning the cultural property of member nations. This and other attempts to stem the tide of illicit trade in antiquities all over the world have also received a good deal of publicity and caught the imagination of the educated and concerned public.

The 1904-1905 excavations at Aphrodisias were inevitably defined by nineteenth-century archaeological practices and standards. They were not aimed, apparently, in any specific direction, except

For years, the people of old Geyre and its surrounding neighbourhood made use of the boxes of sarcophagi from the Roman necropolis that lies all around the walls of the city. Until recently, as this photograph shows, they would press the grapes from the vineyards surrounding the village in these stone coffins occasionally to produce wine, but more frequently to make a type of grape jelly (*pekmez*) by boiling the juice.

towards the exploration (not to say exploitation) of a rich site and the acquisition of works of art and artefacts for private or public collections. The Italian mission of 1937 was too short-lived to reveal clear objectives; it merely carried on in the old inconsistent if profitable tradition. The principle aims of the current project, which is sponsored by New York University, are nevertheless based on the results, however incompletely published, of the work of our predecessors and subsequent research that was based on their discoveries.

One specific objective at the outset of our project was a definition of the vast quantity of sculpture unearthed at the site and apparently created there in Roman times — as some scholars suggest, in the spirit of a 'school' of art.

Survey of the Site

After a preliminary visit to Aphrodisias in 1959, it became obvious that an accurate topographical survey, almost non-existent from previous excavations, should be undertaken first. This should then be followed by a detailed study and inventory of all monumental remains that were visible above ground. Only then would the excavation of selected areas begin.

Once formalities with the Directorate-General of Antiquities and Museums of Turkey were completed and we had been granted permission to start work, we were confronted by several immediate problems. The most frustrating of these was the presence of the village of Geyre, occupying a large portion of the eastern and south-eastern area of the ancient city. A governmental decree in 1956 had resolved to resettle the villagers of Geyre at a site two kilometres to the west, and construction of the new village was proceeding well by 1961. Nevertheless old Geyre continued to be densely populated. Another major obstacle was the fact that most of the site, apart from the areas overlaid by the village houses, consisted of fields and poplar groves not only privately owned but also under cultivation. Only a limited area around the Temple of Aphrodite, the Stadium and the Baths of Hadrian was public land. Inevitably, therefore, our explorations and excavation plans were restricted in their early phases.

Despite these problems, a thorough survey of the ancient city's remains was initiated in 1961. This was completed in subsequent campaigns and was further refined by means of balloon photography in 1977 and 1979.

The slopes of the Baba Dağ range to the east were explored at the same time. It was here, only a few kilometres away from Aphrodisias, that the marble which played such a significant role in the life

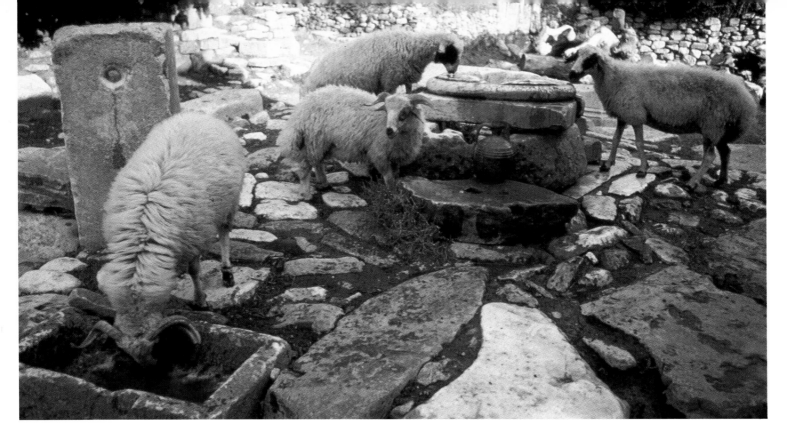

Many architectural fragments were cleverly reused for a variety of purposes, such as well heads or animal drinking troughs (*above*).

After pressing the grapes in sarcophagi, the villagers would collect and filter the extracted juice into large bronze cauldrons (*left*), then boil it to produce *pekmez*, the grape jelly used as a jam or pleasantly flavoured sweetener.

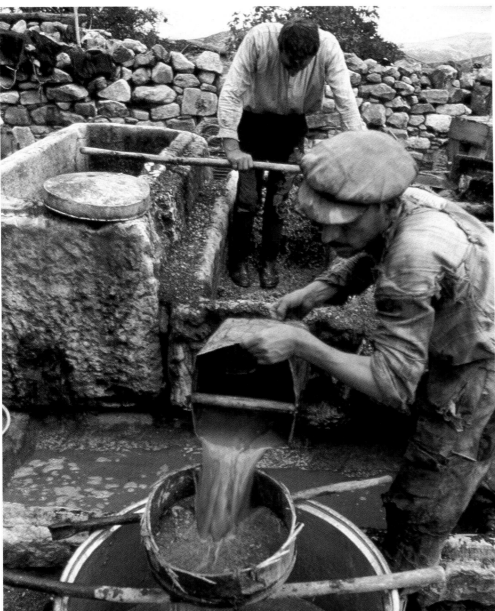

This plan of the site (*opposite*) shows the extent of excavations to date. It is expected that unexcavated areas will eventually yield as many outstanding public and private buildings with their lavish decorations and sculpture, as have been revealed so far.

Today, the archaeologist's responsibility entails protection and restoration of the monuments that he has uncovered as much as scholarly study and publication. In Turkey, restoration activities are a mandatory condition in the terms of the permit issued to anyone who wishes to excavate. The Aphrodisias project has met this requirement as faithfully as possible and especially in recent years has accelerated discrete restoration procedures, or anastylosis, in the more remarkable building complexes that have been brought to light. An example is the Sebasteion, where the lifting of an inscribed architrave block on to the re-erected half-columns of the north portico is shown.

of the city had been found in abundance and quarried. The blocks were cut and worked in the quarry and then conveyed by ox-carts or other means to the Maeander valley and beyond. Exploration revealed over twenty quarrying sites or refuse pits, which contained marble of various grains, often with a grey-blue tint that occasionally developed into dark blue-grey coloured veins.

Aphrodisias is located on an essentially flat portion of a plateau some six hundred metres high, which inclines gently towards the south-west, near the course of the river Geyre. The Geyre's waters, joined by other streams, flow north-westward to form the Dandalas, a tributary of the Maeander. Among these waterways were the ancient Morsynos and Timeles, named on some of the coins of the city and personified as river-gods.

The only topographical irregularity of the site is a hillock of roughly conical shape and about twenty metres in height. Gaudin labelled it the 'Acropolis', without realising that it was one of two artificial mounds, or *höyük*, that formed the core of prehistoric settlements in this region. The second mound, subsequently named '*Pekmez*', was unfortunately in great part obliterated by later habitations. Its name — also given to the area around the mound — comes from the villagers' practice of making a grape jelly or sweetener called *pekmez* here, pressing the fruits in ancient sarcophagi and boiling the resulting mush in large copper cauldrons. Traces of the mound are evident in a slightly more elevated section of the village to the east of the 'Acropolis'.

An elaborate system of fortification walls, with a roughly circular

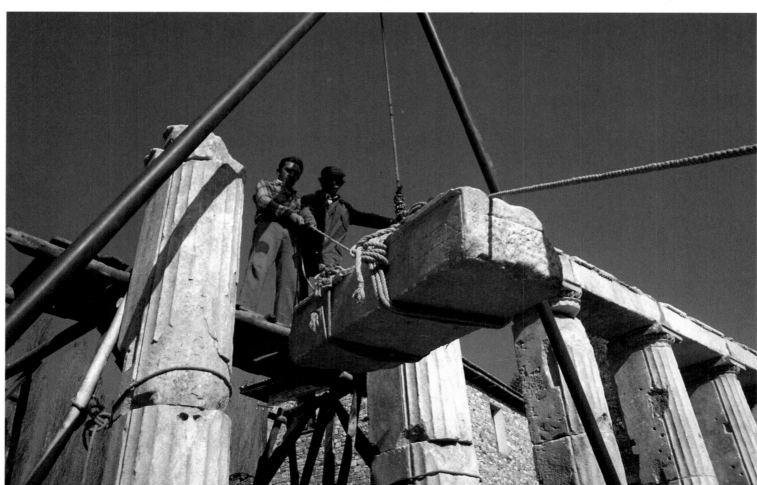

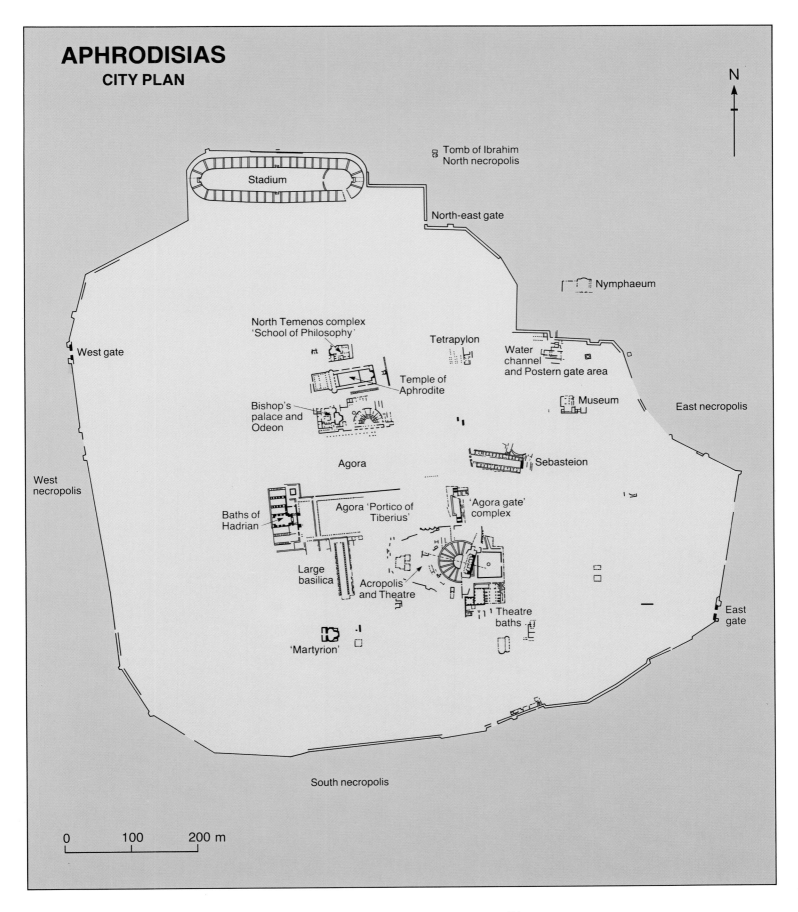

APHRODISIAS
CITY PLAN

N

Stadium

Tomb of Ibrahim
North necropolis

North-east gate

Nymphaeum

North Temenos complex
'School of Philosophy'

Tetrapylon

Water
channel
and Postern gate area

West gate

Temple of
Aphrodite

Bishop's
palace and
Odeon

Museum

East necropolis

Agora

Sebasteion

West
necropolis

Baths of
Hadrian

Agora 'Portico of
Tiberius'

'Agora gate'
complex

Large
basilica

Acropolis
and Theatre

Theatre
baths

East
gate

'Martyrion'

South necropolis

0   100   200 m

perimeter of about three and a half kilometres, encompassed the area of about two hundred and fifty acres that comprised the heart of the ancient city. These fortifications featured, at intervals, a number of towers and at least four principal gates that were located at the cardinal points. Stretches of the walls are preserved almost to their full height in the northern, eastern and western sectors of the circuit. Their southern portions are more collapsed, although their course can be traced.

The construction of these walls reveals the reuse of much architectural, epigraphical and even sculptural material at certain points. There also appear to have been several phases of building and restoration. It is possible that construction began in the late third century AD, when Gothic invasions of the 250s and 260s ravaged or threatened parts of western Anatolia. However, epigraphical evidence seems to point to a systematic building or drastic reworking of the circuit in or shortly after the middle of the fourth century. The reuse of second-hand architectural blocks on a large scale may have occurred in the aftermath of an earthquake, or earthquakes, that damaged the walls and made available material from destroyed buildings, for instance from those in the vicinity of the Theatre. Such catastrophes in the 350s and 360s may well have been responsible for these building and rebuilding activities.

It is difficult to explain the reasons for some of the irregularities in

No clear evidence of a fortification system pre-dating the late third or fourth century AD has so far been detected or uncovered at Aphrodisias. The fragmentary walls often stand to their full height and feature a number of watch towers and traces of 'chemin de ronde'. At least four main gateways cut through this wall at approximately the four cardinal points. The gate shown here faces west and bears an inscription of the fourth century AD; it is referred to as the Antioch Gate, because it leads to the city of Antioch-on-the-Maeander situated to the north-west.

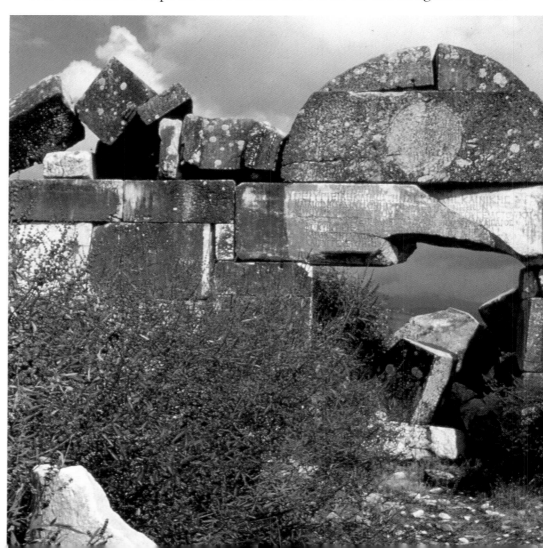

the perimeter walls, although many were probably dictated by the presence of buildings or their remains. It is obvious, for instance, that the large, well-preserved stadium had to be incorporated within the circuit: had it been left out it could have been used by a besieging enemy to mount an attack against the city. Although the area beyond the fortifications consisted of a vast necropolis, there is strong evidence that the city extended there too, as remains of secular, non-funerary buildings have been recorded at several locations outside the walls.

At many points the fortification walls straddle important sepulchral monuments. This occurs especially to the west and the south-east, where the walls incorporate decorative elements and inscriptions within their fabric. A thorough brush-clearing and reinvestigation of the circuit in 1975 brought to light many epigraphic sarcophagus and sculpture fragments, some of them connected with the Archive Wall of the Theatre. Excavations were also undertaken within the inner face of the southern walls. Below the accumulation of architectural debris from the upper courses, a series of early Byzantine dwellings, perhaps guard-houses, were found nestling beside the walls.

Evidence concerning earlier walls or fortification systems is still unclear. It is possible that some defence arrangements existed in the Hellenistic period on or near the 'Acropolis', prior to the construc-

A large number of architectural fragments, inscribed statue bases and other similar remnants are clearly seen in the better preserved portions of the fortification walls such as the northern stretch shown here. These architectural pieces were reused here after the buildings to which they originally belonged were damaged by earthquakes. It is easier to assume such damage than to imagine that, even in the face of great danger, the Aphrodisians would have been willing or even able deliberately to dismantle so many of their buildings to construct or repair their walls.

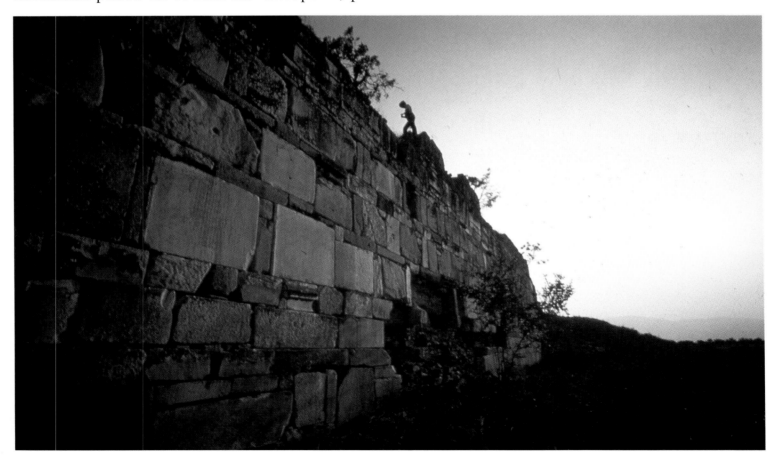

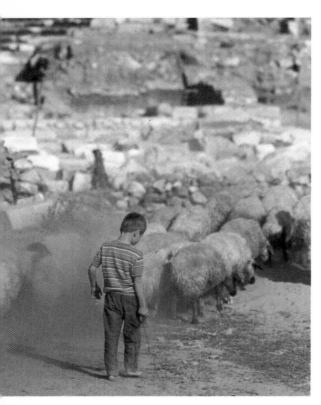

The charm of early work at Aphrodisias was accentuated by the ever-present reminders of simple village life and farming activities. Sadly, with increased mechanization, the pleasant, muted patter of passing sheep and donkeys have inexorably been replaced by the roar and rattle of tractors and their trailers.

tion of the Theatre on its eastern slope. Indeed, certain massive buttressed constructions found there do not seem to be part of the substructures of the Theatre. If this is evidence of an older fortification system, such an arrangement would provide an earlier parallel to the later, seventh-century transformation of the 'Acropolis' into a citadel, which made free use of architectural material from nearby buildings damaged by earthquake.

The Temple of Aphrodite

The main excavation activities of our annual campaigns in the 1960s concentrated on the Temple of Aphrodite. This building is one of the major sacred structures of western Asia Minor and unquestionably merited our full attention. Unfortunately, the extensive remodellings to which it had been subjected during its transformation into a Christian basilica tend to obscure its earlier features. Although duly reported in words and drawings by the Society of Dilettanti and others, its remains had never been properly analysed. On circumstantial evidence, it had been dated to the reign of the Emperor Hadrian (117-138).

The objectives of our early operations here included obtaining a better understanding of the sequence of building and rebuilding, as well as exploring possible antecedents and looking for specific details of its conversion into a Christian church. The haphazard trenches and dumps left by Gaudin were still visible among piles of architectural *disiecta membra* accumulated in the nave of the basilica. Despite this state of disarray, fourteen columns of the peristyle of the Temple still stood, battered but erect, like wounded sentinels of Aphrodite's shrine.

Before investigating the pagan sanctuary proper, we aimed to define or verify the remodelling work accomplished by the Byzantine architects. We noted the presence of a corner Ionic capital on the penultimate column of the north peristyle and another one on the eighth column, from the west, of the south peristyle. This suggested that the early Christian rebuilders had probably left these colonnades of the temple in place, but had moved the columns of the east and west ends in order to extend those of the long north and south sides. Their ultimate purpose was to transform the building into a basilica — that is to say a structure with a central nave flanked by two aisles. Two walls were added to the north and south, parallel to the colonnades, in order to frame the aisles. The area to the east was filled in to allow the construction of an apse and two dependencies on either side (a diakonikon and prothesis).

These alterations were naturally influenced by various features of the pagan temple; especially its temenos, or sacred precinct, which

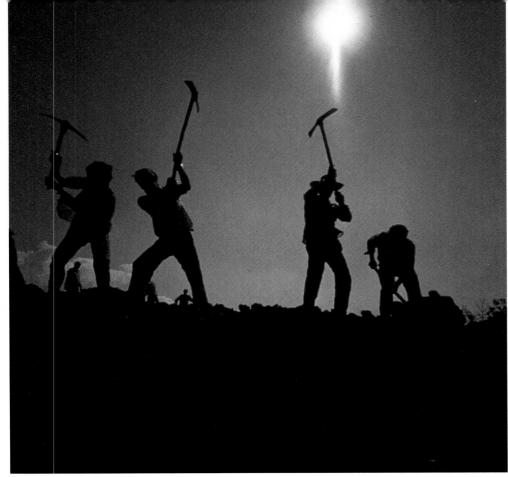

Much credit for the amazing amount of discoveries made at Aphrodisias must be given to the hard work of our dedicated and loyal workmen who hail from new Geyre and its neighbouring villages.

Despite the depredations of time, nature and the hand of man, the precinct and the Temple of Aphrodite remains the most evocative central point of the ruined city. In the late afternoon, as the sun sets, its wounded columns and guardian lion are silhouetted against the eastern sky, and provide a dramatic frame for cloud-topped Baba Dağ on the horizon.

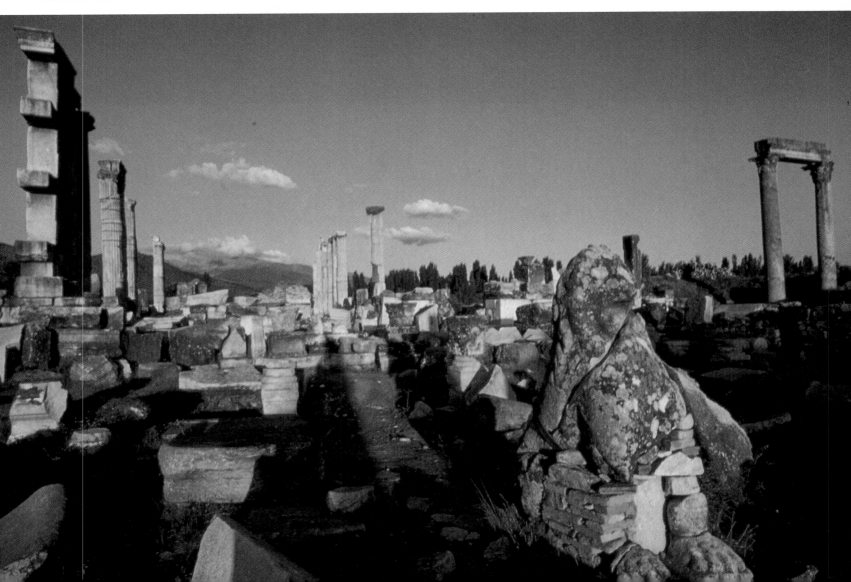

surround the sanctuary. According to available evidence, mainly based on measurements and the assumption that the corner Ionic capitals had remained *in situ*, the temple was octastyle, had thirteen columns on its long sides, and faced east. It appears to have had an altar arrangement or an earlier temenos wall, which the Byzantine architects decided to make use of for backing the apse of their basilica.

There was, however, a much more ornate temenos of later date, which, according to epigraphic evidence, was clearly Hadrianic. It consisted of a series of niches (aediculae or naiskoi), framed by Corinthian columns, on all four sides of the temple. The eastern columns of this temenos were incorporated by the Byzantines into a double narthex system giving access to the church. Beyond this, an atrium or entrance court, as well as a small baptistery, were added to the west.

The interior walls of the pagan shrine proper (the cella or naos) were completely levelled to the ground and some of their blocks re-used in the construction of the aisle walls to the north and south. The Christian altar area included a bema, an iconostasis (sanctuary screen) and a ciborium (canopy arrangement) in front of the apse, at the eastern end of the nave. The ciborium stood by a sacred well before a synthronon: a semicircular seating area for the bishop of Aphrodisias and other church officials.

It is possible that the well in question was originally the pagan one

Investigations of the Temple of Aphrodite, which was originally completed in the late first century BC, were much hampered by drastic but clever transformations of its design (in the late fifth century AD) into that of a Christian basilica. Following serious earthquake damage in the seventh century AD the church was partly repaired in the eleventh or twelfth century AD. Its final demise occurred soon afterward, however, at the hands of Seljuk and Turkoman raiders.

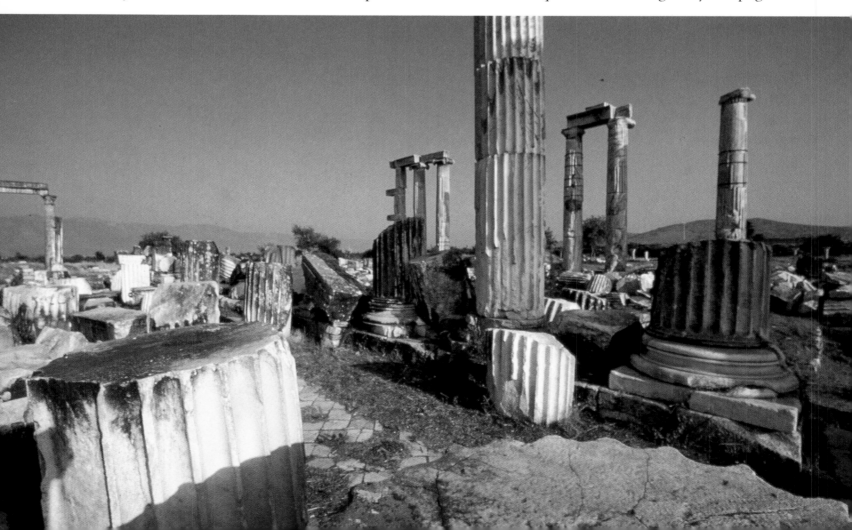

mentioned by the second-century travel writer, Pausanias (I. 26.5). This would have been cleaned and consecrated by the Christian builders. A semicircular covered passageway was discovered between the synthronon and the wall of the apse. Traces of frescoes on its walls, showing parts of a seated Christ, the Virgin, and saints, appear to date from between the tenth and twelfth centuries. There is also evidence of remodelling in the church at about this time, perhaps following damage or destruction.

Regarding the date of the original major work to convert the pagan shrine into the Christian church, evidence points to the fifth century. The basilica was apparently dedicated to Saint Michael, and its consecration might have taken place in 443 and been associated with a visit by the emperor Theodosius II. Unfortunately, all these Byzantine innovations, including the later building of a few tombs inside the basilica and a larger cemetery outside, considerably upset the stratigraphy relating to the pagan temple, and confused much of the archaeological material.

A number of soundings have provided evidence that establishes a date for the building of the pagan temple in the first century BC (and not one in the second century AD as formerly supposed). This had, indeed, already been suggested by several stylistic aspects of its architecture.

The Temple's construction may actually have begun earlier than this date, before being interrupted or damaged during the turbulent years of the Second Triumvirate. It was, however, surely completed during the reign of Augustus. The interior arrangement of the pagan sanctuary was partly revealed by a series of small trenches, difficult to dig and interpret. The foundations of the cella and a pronaos were also brought to light. Thus the inner sanctum of the Temple, where the image of the goddess was kept, was seen to have consisted of a large chamber preceded by a porch or pronaos. Apparently there was no opisthodomos, or treasury-room, behind the cella, although traces of some foundations of uncertain purpose survive at this point. On the other hand, the foundations of the pronaos seemed to break through the remains of a mosaic floor, made of crude tesserae, which included traces of blue-black borderlines against a white background, and animal figures in an emblema, or separated area.

This mosaic probably pertained to a pre-first century BC building which, because of the sacred nature of the spot, should logically be connected with a temple or sanctuary. A date for the floor (and by implication the building it once decorated) was provided by three coins of the early third century BC found embedded in its mortar during the removal and conservation of its fragments. However, the precise relationship of this evidence to other traces of foundations remains problematic because of a series of levelling operations and removals of foundation stones during the construction of the first-century BC temple, and as a result of Byzantine conversion. Indeed, soundings dug in front of the pronaos presented several problems of

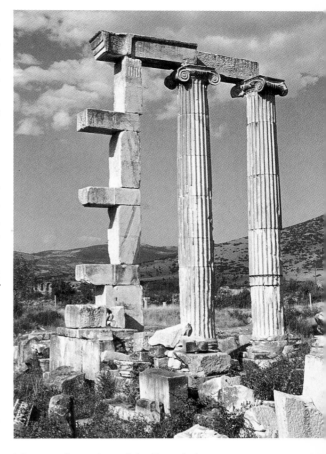

The transformation of the Temple into a Christian basilica involved the complete uprooting of the large blocks of the shrine or cella, which was the repository of the cult statue. A number of the Ionic columns originally surrounding the cella were moved and re-erected to create the basilica plan. A number of cella blocks were aligned at the west end of the new basilica with side columns to join them to a newly created narthex. This gives an unexpected, but now characteristic, silhouette to the north-west corner of the basilica.

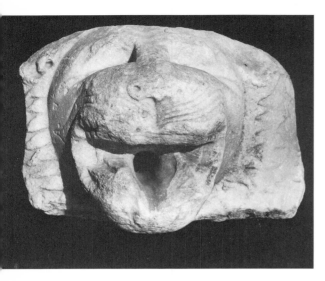

Clear testimony in the form of pottery and terracotta figurine fragments betrays the existence of an archaic shrine to Aphrodite at or near the site of the first-century BC temple. The only architectural evidence datable to the later sixth century BC, however, is a gutter spout in the shape of a lion's head. Unfortunately, this fragment was found by Gaudin in 1904 and is imprecisely documented except for the mention of its discovery 'near the Temple of Aphrodite'. No other architectural element of clear archaic date has yet been located by the present excavations, although the lion-spout in question undoubtedly belonged to a building of some size. It is probable that many if not most of the stones of such an earlier shrine were reused or recarved in the course of the building of the first-century BC temple.

interpretation, some of these due to the discovery of traces of stone packing of uncertain date, while deeper probes produced fragmentary walls that may have acted as foundations or supports. Some of them must be of archaic date, to judge from the potsherds recovered. Yet, later Hellenistic material was also mixed with these sherds.

The existence of an archaic temple was already implied by a lion-spout found in 1904 by Gaudin, which must have belonged to a building of some size. However, the lack of precise information in Gaudin's notes concerning the discovery of this fragment, as well as limited additional architectural evidence, prevented definite conclusions from being drawn regarding the archaic shrine. On the other hand, three fragmentary terracotta figurines of a seated goddess of the sixth century BC were discovered in a trench behind the apse of the church, unfortunately, once again in a disturbed context. These support the evidence for the lion-spout belonging to an early or archaic phase in the history of the cult of the divinity. Regrettably, the frequent building, rebuilding and levelling activities, as well as the reuse of some earlier material in the Temple area, led to constant churning and mixing and eventual obliteration of a clear stratigraphy. Nevertheless, additional material is constantly being unearthed, and many areas area still to be explored fully, so the search for a clearer picture of the various phases of the temple has not yet been abandoned.

By a remarkable stroke of good fortune, three fragments of a colossal marble statue of Aphrodite were found in 1962 immediately south of the temenos. They had been incorporated into the foundations of a later wall. The face and arms of the goddess had been mutilated by pious Christian hands, but the figure could still be restored. The patron divinity of the city was represented fully dressed in a long characteristic outer garment, or *ependytes*. This was horizontally divided into relief-decorated panels featuring the Three Graces. These were flanked by the busts of Hera and Zeus; followed by those of Selene (the Moon) and Helios (the Sun); then by Aphrodite herself riding over the sea on Capricorn guided by a winged Triton and followed by a dolphin; and, finally, by three Erotes performing a sacrifice at an altar. This statue had almost certainly been dragged from the Temple area by the Byzantines and buried nearby. It is unlikely, however, that it is the cult-statue itself, since that holy image was likely to have been made of more precious material and stones.

Many smaller replicas of this figure have been found in several parts of the Mediterranean, and are particularly numerous in Rome. These were probably taken along by travellers, pilgrims, and itinerant citizens of Aphrodisias. It is reasonable to suppose that a significant proportion of the latter would have been Aphrodisian sculptors called away by commissions, or travelling in search of employment.

This image of the goddess, who symbolised fertility and life, also reflects her embodiment of the forces of nature. She reigned supreme not only over heaven and the underworld, but also over the sea and earth. The figure echoes other Anatolian nature- and mother-goddesses of local or widespread fame, such as the Artemis of Ephesus. Scholars generally agree that such representations are creations of the Hellenistic period, replacing earlier, more primitive, idol-like sacred images of great antiquity.

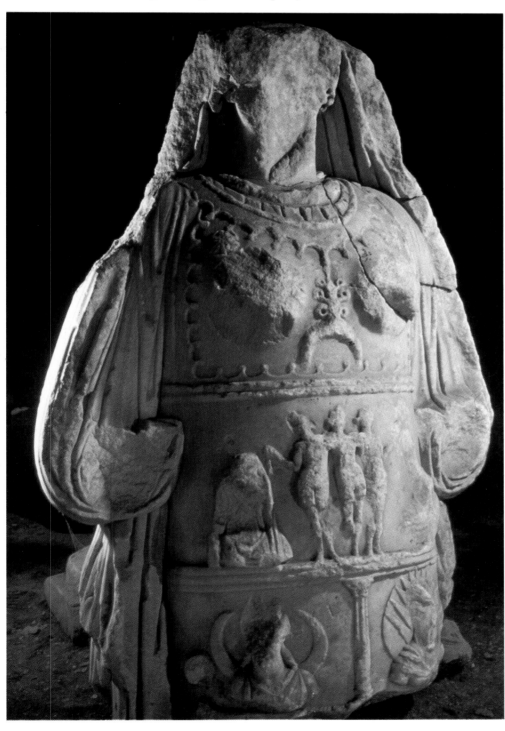

Pious Christian hands mutilated the upper torso of the colossal image of the goddess of the city. This fragment, together with its lower portion, were accidentally recovered in 1962 in a Byzantine foundation wall to the south of the precinct of Aphrodite. This statue would have stood inside that precinct. The cult statue itself, safeguarded in the cella, was probably made of more precious and delicate materials and so would have been completely destroyed by the early Christians. The goddess of Aphrodisias symbolized all forms of life and fertility in the universe, as indicated in the registers shown in relief on her elaborately decorated and close-fitting tunic. Although battered, the representations of The Three Graces, flanked by busts of Hera and Zeus, and above other busts of Selene, the moon, and Helios, the sun, are identifiable.

The Tetrapylon

Among the most attractive landmarks of the ruins of Aphrodisias, at the western entrance to Geyre, is a pair of spirally fluted Corinthian columns topped by an architrave block and facing the Temple to the west. Their elegant and decorative beauty, enhanced by the swaying poplar groves behind them to the south, delighted many an early traveller and have frequently provided inspiration for photographers in our own day.

Excavations, followed by temporary restoration, were undertaken here in 1963 and revealed that the columns formed part of an elaborately decorated monumental gateway. As it included four rows of four columns, it came to be known as the Tetrapylon. Its specific relationship to the temenos of Aphrodite, some hundred metres to the west, is not clear because another entrance, or propylon, gave access to the Temple through the temenos wall. However, some of its stylistic peculiarities suggest that it was built more or less at the same time as the temenos, about the middle of the second century AD or shortly thereafter.

In 1970, a careful review of all the recovered architectural elements by one of our collaborators, Dr Alois Machatschek of Vienna, resulted in a series of handsome restoration drawings as well as a better appreciation of the building. These show that the Tetrapylon consisted of four rows of four columns placed on high bases. From the east, the first and third rows were spirally fluted, while the shafts of the columns of the fourth row were smooth. The

The remaining columns of the Tetrapylon, seen from the east looking west and including the elegantly spirally fluted columns of the east façade frame the Temple of Aphrodite in the distance. This delicately conceived decorative gateway acted as an attractive access to the precinct of Aphrodite. It was flanked by a recently uncovered and evidently important well-paved street running roughly north-south toward the Sebasteion and the Theatre. Extensive restoration of the gateway is being currently undertaken following intensive study and architectural evaluation.

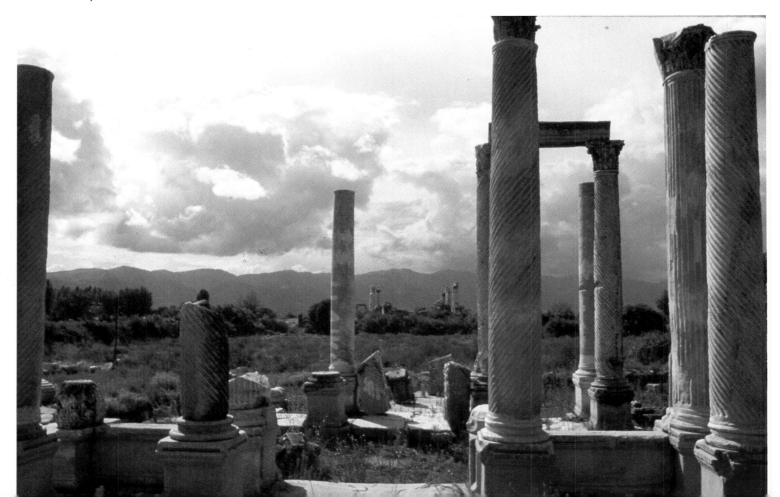

second row columns, on the other hand, were double as their intercolumniations were apparently closed by marble lattice-work screens.

The access side, and the main façade of the Tetrapylon, was to the east; the first row of spirally-fluted columns acted as a decorative front. The gateway also served as a sort of crossway, since a paved road passed in the wider interval between the second and third rows running approximately north to south. A highly decorative broken pediment with a curved lintel featured between the second and third columns of the first row and was echoed by a semicircular lunette on the second row. A similar arrangement was conceived on the west, or temple side of the gateway. The sides of the broken pediment were lavishly and exuberantly adorned with relief figures of Nikes (at the corners) and Erotes hunting wild boars and stags with dogs. These and additional rich angle decorations must have provoked the admiration of many visitors to the city of Aphrodisias. Even in their ruined condition they are still able to enchant us today.

The presence of several village houses nearby, and the passage of the road connecting old Geyre with the new village, unfortunately hindered our work here in the 1970s. More recently, however, the expropriation and removal of the houses and elimination of the roadway enabled us to resume work on the Tetrapylon. In 1984 we began to restore it in a discreet fashion, on the basis of previous studies, with the aim of revealing more than the present mere hint of its former beauty.

The western façade of the Tetrapylon, facing the Temple, presents four rows of smooth Corinthian columns topped by an exuberantly decorated broken pediment *(below left and centre)* featuring beguiling figures of mounted or running Erotes and elegant Nikes rising from richly curling acanthus leaves. Hidden among these are animals such as the wild boar *(below right)* which suggests that these are depictions of hunting scenes.

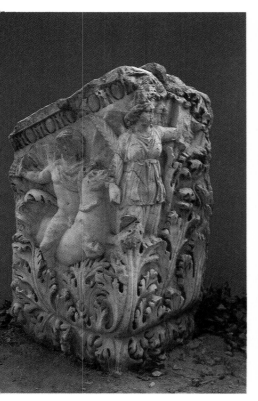

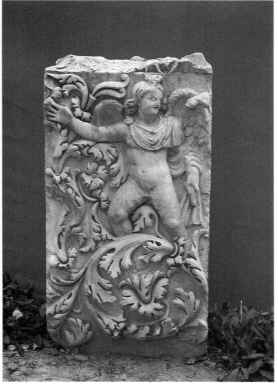

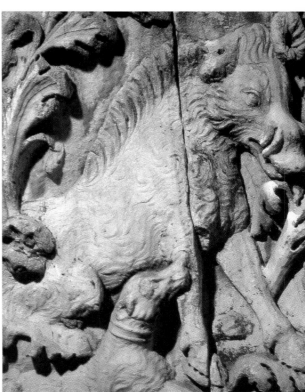

The Odeon, and a Sculptor's Workshop

One of our major discoveries in 1962 seemed to be prompted by Aphrodite herself. Immediately to the south of the Temple, a continuation of the exploratory trench that had brought to light the fragments of the colossal cult-statue of Aphrodite, reached a slight depression. This had been planted with the remains of a lentil crop, and lay at the edge of the agora of the city. Further trenching revealed an extremely well-preserved series of semicircular tiers of seats. Expropriative measures were rapidly undertaken in 1963 and, in subsequent years, a small, gem-like theatrical structure, or Odeon, was slowly excavated.

Like many other buildings at Aphrodisias, the Odeon was decorated with ultimate refinement in its details. Its surviving cavea consists of nine rows of elegant seats, divided into five sectors or cunei, the ends adorned with lions' legs. The discovery of interconnected supporting chambers and elaborate sub-structures below and behind the cavea clearly suggest that the Odeon was once roofed and included an upper section. The idea that there had been a roof was reinforced by the presence of supporting pillars placed at intervals on the building's semicircular outer rim.

In its original roofed condition the seating capacity of the Odeon was probably about 1,700 spectators. Presumably the roof or the upper section — or both — were seriously damaged in one of the

One of the architectural gems of Aphrodisias, the Odeon, is especially appealing in the late afternoon, when its remaining tiers of marble seats glow warmly in the soft light of the setting sun. This effect could not, however, have been appreciated when the building was still in its original form, for it then would not only have had an upper series of seats, but also would have been surrounded by walls and completely covered by a roof *(see reconstruction drawing in appendix)*. The semicircular orchestra of the Odeon was paved with multicoloured opus sectile mosaic *(opposite below)*. It seems likely the flooding occurred after earthquake damage in the later fourth century.

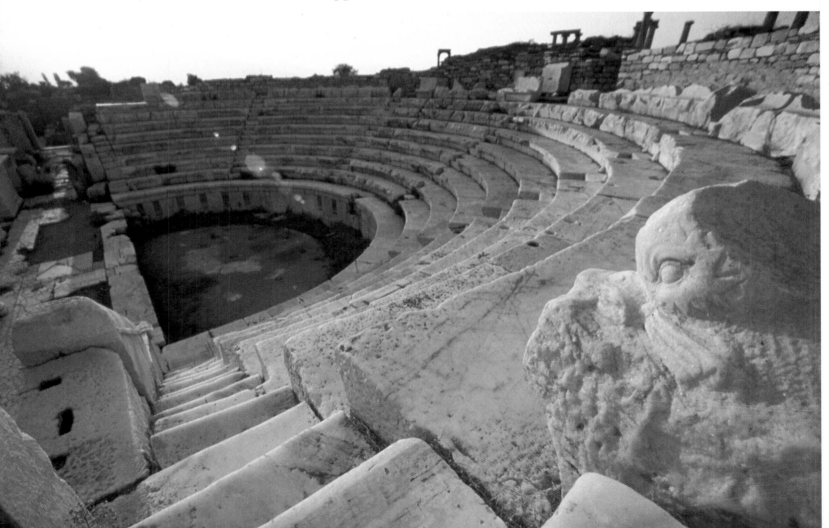

earthquakes of the fourth century. Thereafter the Odeon was perhaps used open to the sky. A lovely multicoloured mosaic of the opus sectile type, featuring white and dark-blue marble, together with red slate lozenges and squares, decorated the deep orchestra floor, but did not reach the edge of the cavea.

It seems that at least one row of seats had been removed to give depth to the semicircular orchestra, while steps had been added in the centre of the cavea and on either side to permit descent from the stage into the orchestra pit. These alterations may have been due to functional changes, but were more probably dictated by the need to control seeping underground waters, which could have been released by one of the fourth-century earthquakes. As in a number of other low-lying areas of the city, especially in the vicinity of the Agora, these problems due to water infiltration afflicted the Odeon occasionally. Even in recent years its orchestra pit has been filled, to the great delight of the local frog and terrapin population.

The stage of the Odeon contained elaborately decorated, high bases supporting architectural niches (naiskoi or aediculae) in which handsome statuary was placed. Among the sculptures recovered there are exquisitely carved figures of seated poets or philosophers, as well as full-length portraits of high officials and symbolic representations of the city's governing institutions.

The performances here would have been on a small and intimate scale — musical comedies, ballets, pantomimes and, of course,

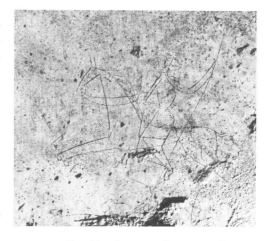

Many graffiti, like this one of a mounted horseman, have been found in the backstage corridor of the Odeon.

The repairs to reduce the problem of flooding seem to have consisted of the removal of the front rows of seats of the lower cavea, which created a semicircular strip in the orchestra area in which water could collect. To this day water still seeps into the orchestra, the quantity depending on the winter and spring rains. Taking advantage of drier summer conditions *(below right)*, the mosaic floor was duly cleaned and removed for safety, preservation and eventual display.

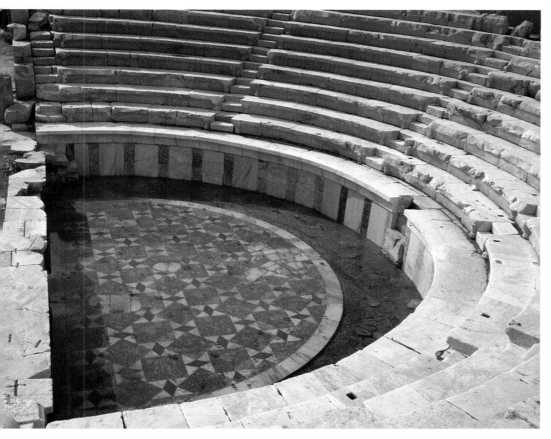

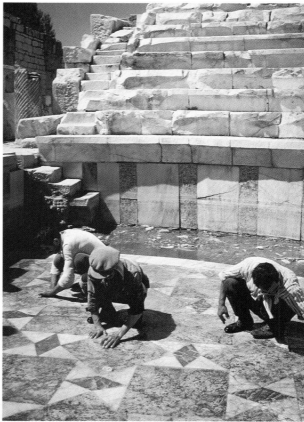

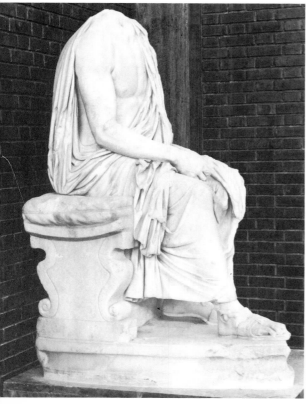

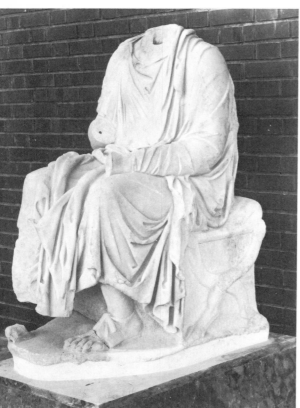

Two statues of seated poets or philosophers that once decorated the stage of the Odeon.

concerts. Lectures, political discussions and administrative meetings involving the local senate or the city council must also have taken place here, making full use of the auditorium's facilities. It is known that other theatres were frequently used for larger political gatherings, and the location of the Odeon, facing the public area or agora of the city, clearly suggests its suitability for use in the city's public affairs.

In 1965, a portico was excavated behind the stage corridor. It consisted of interior Corinthian columns and external Ionic columns facing the Agora, with unfluted lower drums similar to those still standing in parts of the market place. Several portrait statues, particularly two late second-century representations of the Aphrodisian notables L. Ant. Dometinus Diogenes and apparently his wife, Claudia Antonia Tatiana, were recovered from where they had fallen in front of their inscribed bases. Both Diogenes and Tatiana wore diadems or head-dresses decorated with the bust of Aphrodite in the centre and around her, those of emperors and empresses whose cult was associated with that of the goddess of the city.

In the back-stage corridor of the Odeon, more intimate inscriptions were found: the plaster of the walls was covered with graffiti, scratched caricatures and imprecations, giving evidence of the foibles, fancies and minor forms of self-expression of later Aphrodisians.

A date in the late first or second century for the construction of the Odeon can be inferred from a preliminary study of its architectural decoration. It is also possible that a gymnasium-type complex may have been located in this area south of the Temple of Aphrodite before that time. Traces of it were detected in exploratory trenches behind and to the west of the supporting chambers of the collapsed summa cavea. A monument was also found here, which may have been associated with this gymnasium. It consisted of a well-built, circular platform of three steps, and was partly covered by the Odeon walls to the north-west of the building. On the platform were the remains of polygonal shapes decorated with finely modelled lions' feet. Inside was a sarcophagus with roughly cut garland designs on its sides and a flat lid, almost certainly thrown aside by looters at a later date. Nestled against the stone coffin was a circular altar, finely decorated with beguiling figures of smiling Erotes supporting beribboned garlands of fruit and flowers. This monument must have been the final resting place (or *heroon*) of an important individual in the first century, as, in classical times, only notables were allowed to be interred within the confines of the city.

In the late Roman and early Byzantine period, especially after the fourth-century earthquakes, this whole area (as well as the back chambers of the Odeon) was used for a while for the production of wine and olive oil. Numerous large, marble storage jars, or *pithoi*, and parts of wine or olive presses were discovered strewn about. Immediately to the south of the temenos of Aphrodite many trial pieces or half finished or discarded sculptures were also recorded in the course of excavations.

More extensive investigations brought to light at least two chambers where such debris was concentrated. In these chambers, three iron punches that were used for carving marble were also found. The identification of a sculptor's workshop area here under the aegis, as it were, of Aphrodite herself, is further aided by the discovery of abundant 'pockets' of marble chips in the stratigraphy of trenches near the rooms. The workshop appears to have been destroyed in the late fourth century. Its contents were probably scattered about or reused in makeshift walls after one of the earthquakes of the 350s or 360s. Because of the changes in the ground water table and the resultant flooding, the level of the workshop area was raised and a series of water-channels and terracotta pipes were installed in an attempt to evacuate the infiltrating waters.

The discarded and unfinished sculpture pieces associated with the workshop included two versions, one lifesize, the other small, of a figure of a satyr playing with the child Dionysus who is perched on his left shoulder. This subject was recognized due to a partly preserved specimen signed by an Aphrodisian sculptor named Flavius Zenon which was found in Rome, near the Esquiline, in the 1880s. Other items included a well-modelled youthful Herakles; a small

Among the statues adorning the portico behind the Odeon stage facing the Agora, were these two impressive full portraits *(below left and centre)* of Claudia Antonia Tatiana and her husband L. Ant. Dometinus Diogenes, members of Aphrodisian aristocratic society in the late second century AD. Diogenes' head-dress consists of a turban-like arrangement topped by busts, the central one being of Aphrodite. These indicate that his high position included the priesthood of the goddess. The extraordinary achievements in Aphrodisian portrait sculpture are well exemplified in the compelling characterization of Diogenes' face *(below)*.

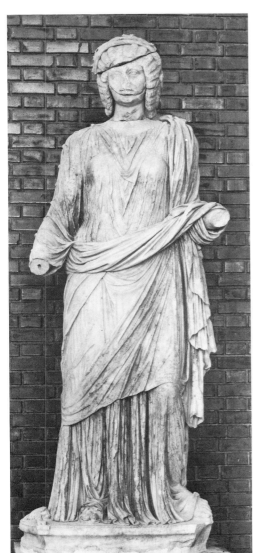
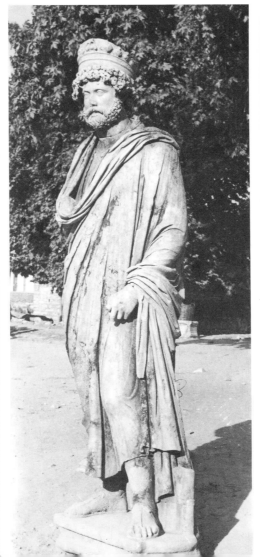
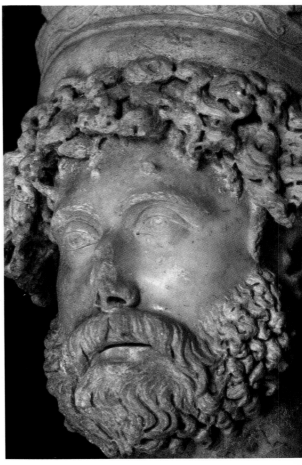

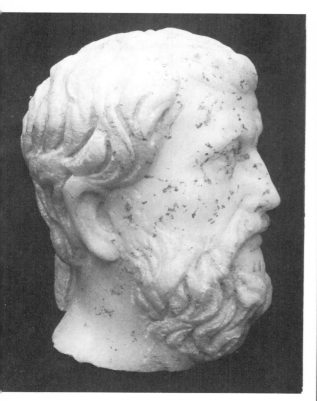

The discovery of the workshop area between the Odeon and the Temple has provided many insights into the production, training, unusual craftsmanship and remarkable aspirations of Aphrodisian sculptors. Two of the most outstanding pieces recovered here are the almost translucent, small portrait head of a philosopher *(above)* dateable to the late second or early third century AD, and the exquisitely modelled, muscular, youthful Herakles *(right)* of approximately the same date.

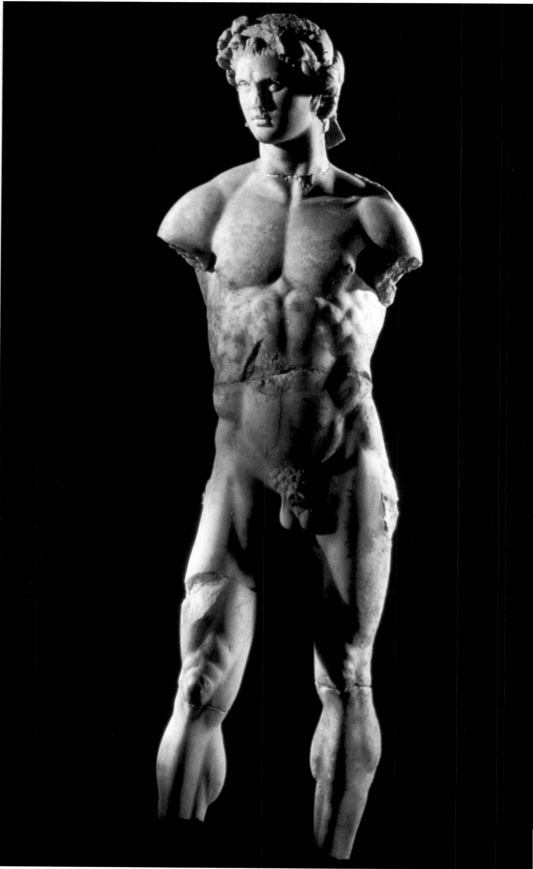

Artemis; and an unfinished 'tour-de-force' figure of Europa seated on Zeus' bull, cunningly carved out of a part white, part blue marble block. There was also an especially intriguing 'reject' statue of a fourth-century official, whose portrait head was incomplete, although the body was smoothly finished. Many other completed and sometimes occasionally highly polished fragments of small sculptures were also found in or near the workshop, and they testify to the production and storage of such material there. Among them, an intact, exquisitely finished, small bearded head is particularly worthy of admiration.

This workshop was only one among many that existed in and near the city. It is reasonable to assume that much of the initial preparation of the blocks to be carved was done near the quarries themselves, leaving the finishing and more refined work to be undertaken in town.

The Stadium

To most early travellers in western Asia Minor, as well as to more recent visitors, the most impressive monument at Aphrodisias was undoubtedly its huge stadium. Even today, despite the rich array of other remains and a treasure-filled museum collection to view, it is hard not to be awestruck by the grandeur of this amazing structure.

It is certainly one of the best preserved of its kind anywhere around the Mediterranean. Consequently, although no excavations were planned, the Stadium was logically one of the first monuments to be included in the initial survey carried out in 1961. It was located in the northern section of the site and was eventually cleverly incorporated into the fortification system. The fortification walls closed the structure's long northern side and its two curved east and west ends, and included a 'curtain' of arcaded recesses above the north-east section. The western barrel-vaulted access passage to the track was entirely blocked by the walls. The eastern one, however, was left open and may have been used as a subsidiary gate or a checkpoint for people entering the city from the north-east. Traces of a further barrel-vaulted access from the city side to the south, were visible near the east end, but the here tiers of seats had either collapsed or been ripped out.

The Stadium includes about thirty tiers of seats and terminates in two semicircular ends to the east and west. It is two hundred and sixty-two metres long and about fifty-nine metres across at its widest point. The long sides are not parallel to one another, but bulge gently toward the middle, giving the track a slightly elliptical shape. Early visitors, like the Society of Dilettanti and others, assumed that this shape was the result of collapse or settling of the seats on these long sides and restored them as parallel in their draw-

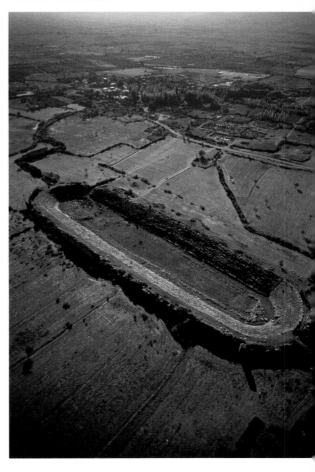

Seen from the air one can easily appreciate why the Stadium is the most stunning monument of Aphrodisias. It is also the best preserved structure of this type in the whole Mediterranean basin.

ings. A more probable explanation is that the elliptical shape reflects optical or viewing considerations. If spectators are seated next to one another in long straight rows they may obstruct each other's view. A slightly curved shape reduces this problem.

From calculations, it seems the Stadium could hold almost 30,000 spectators. It was probably built in the first or second century and would have been used mainly for athletic events and games. It must also have been used for other functions requiring adequate assembly space, such as festivals or public meetings.

Sometime in the Byzantine period, the east end was converted into an area resembling a more typical small arena. Protective walls were added before the lowest row of seats and at least two 'cubicles' or refuges were added to the north edge of the arena. These changes suggest that gladiatorial shows and animal exhibitions were held here, just as they were in the Theatre after the transformations of the second century. The reason for the conversion of the Stadium for

All early travellers record the amazing impression made upon them by the Aphrodisias Stadium, although the structure was heavily overgrown with bushes and trees until the recent excavations. Calculations estimate a capacity of about 30,000 spectators. Today, however, the only spectators are occasional groups of tourists, although the seats remain the favourite haunt of local shepherd boys and their flocks of sheep and goats. The long sides of the Stadium appear to have been purposefully constructed to converge slightly toward each end: this would afford the best possible view for all.

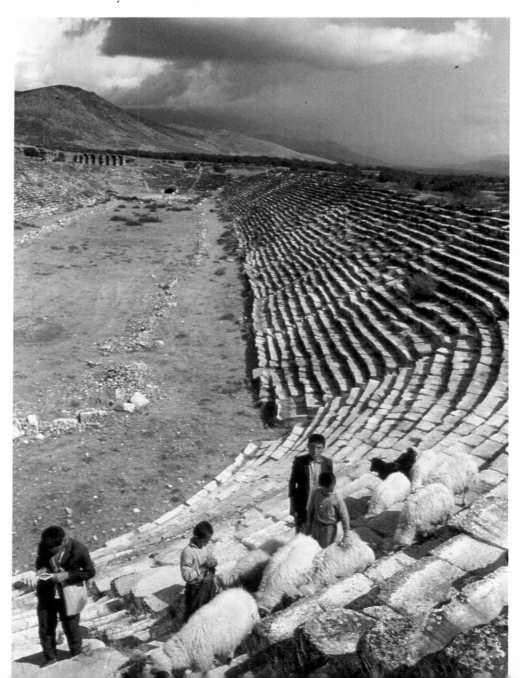

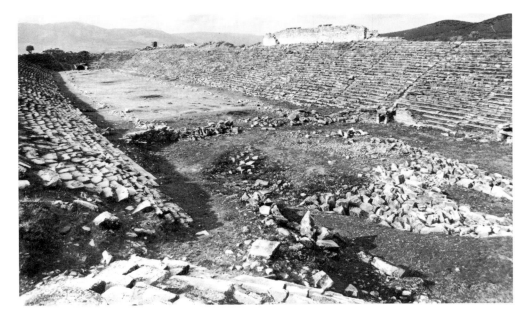

The eastern end of the Stadium was converted into an arena in which to hold circus entertainments, in the modern sense. This probably followed a disastrous seventh-century AD earthquake that rendered unusable the Theatre of the city, which would normally have accommodated such performances.

Four young Turkish wrestlers briefly recreate a scene that illustrates the chief purpose of the Stadium, which was to hold athletic contests and events. These would have included running, jumping, discus and javelin throwing, boxing, and wrestling. It was of course the general convention for participating athletes to perform naked.

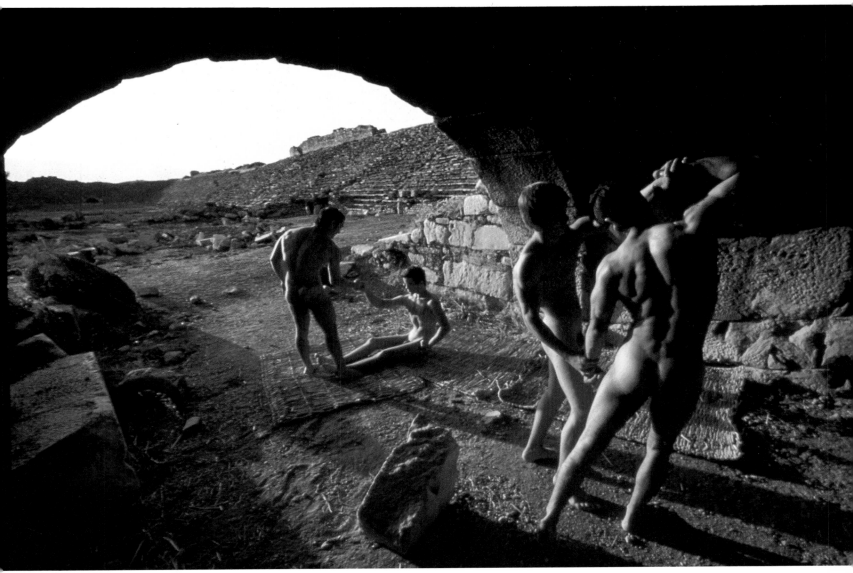

such purposes may be related to the collapse of part of the Theatre, caused by the serious earthquake of the seventh century. It is indeed highly unlikely that Aphrodisias needed two such entertainment arenas at this time.

No work has been attempted in the Stadium during the last twenty campaigns, apart from annual, laborious 'weeding' operations and a small sounding aimed at investigating one of the protruding arches visible along the long southern side. This did not produce any clear results and was therefore discontinued.

There are, of course, many interesting aspects of the Stadium and the activities that took place there that require more detailed examination. Notable among these are the starting lines and some structural peculiarities. Furthermore, the track area would certainly benefit from additional clearing and digging aimed at reaching the ancient level. Such an enterprise would be both costly and time-consuming, however, and would probably yield less information of outstanding importance than excavations elsewhere at Aphrodisias. Therefore, for the time being such work must be deferred.

Roman and Byzantine Residences

One of the most unusual, though by no means unique, facets of Aphrodisias is the opportunity it provides to study the transformation of a prosperous Roman city into a Byzantine town.

The village of Geyre has never occupied more than a modest portion of the ancient site. Most of the buildings over which the stone cottages were built had already been demolished by earthquakes, damaged by other calamities, or buried by their own debris and the silt washed down from the mountain slopes. Furthermore, the lack of substantial urban development in the Ottoman centuries here allows many insights into the life of an eastern Mediterranean provincial city in the Middle Ages.

Excavation and study of the temple of Aphrodite and the Odeon, and of the history of their eventual conversion into buildings with different functions, reveal the ever-present background of the 'classical' Roman past in the life of the Byzantine city. In other words, whether named Aphrodisias, Stavropolis or Caria, the city or town retained something of the appearance of a Roman city, albeit in a state of steady decline, long after Roman influence had dwindled to vanishing point.

This trend was especially obvious after the seventh century, yet the strong classical traditions remained in evidence. The building techniques of Byzantine masons did not radically change from late antiquity onward — nor for that matter did those of their followers, the Turkish inhabitants of Geyre. After the sixth century, however, the skill and expertise of the Aphrodisian sculptors, marble carvers and monumental architects disappeared. This is not surprising since the more plastic arts never played a great part in Byzantine cultural achievements.

The identification of what may have been a palatial residential complex to the south-west of the temple of Aphrodite illustrates, in a private, domestic context, many aspects of the gradual transformation of Aphrodisias from a Roman to a Byzantine city. Discoveries made in the area between the Temple and the Odeon led to additional investigations of remains visible above ground, especially to the west of the Odeon complex. Following expropriation of the land in question, a sizeable building was brought to light.

The building's most striking feature proved to be a triconch hall entered through a large central doorway from an attractive peristyle court. The latter was decorated with blue marble columns on high bases, several of which were eventually re-erected, on the north and east stylobate. Three well-preserved, vaulted chambers of a later

The marble stones of Aphrodisias' monuments glow in the early morning light. To the north of the curtain of poplar trees in the foreground, lie the remains of a luxurious residential complex, perhaps once the palace of a high official or subsequently of the bishop of the city. To the right of this complex can be seen the crescent seating arrangement of the Odeon. Beyond it in the centre of the picture are the pillars of the Temple of Aphrodite, and the Christian basilica that replaced it. Other visible monuments include the Stadium in the distance on the left, and the cluster of columns of the Tetrapylon situated almost due east of the Temple at the edge of the village of old Geyre.

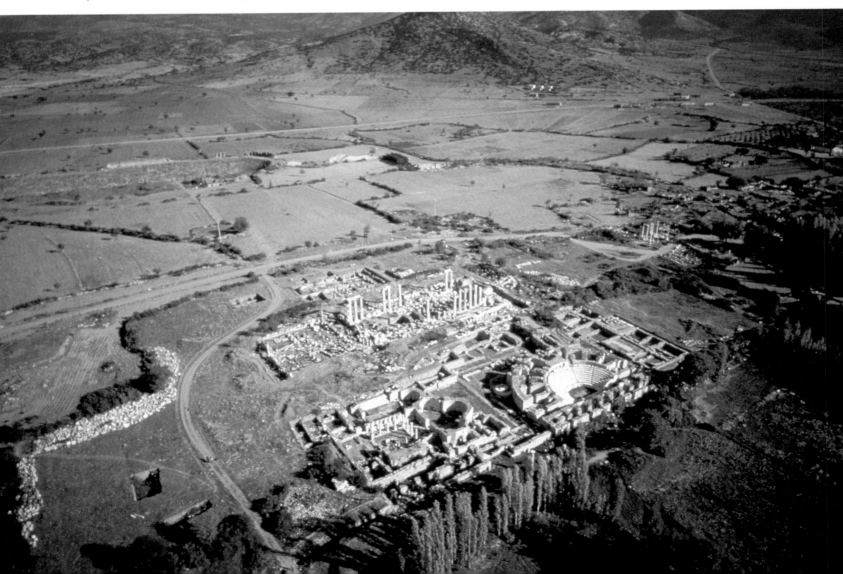

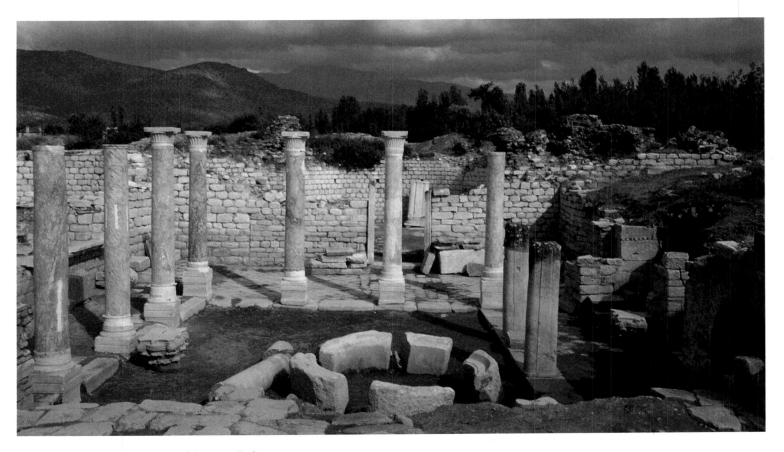

One of the attractive elements of the so-called bishop's palace is a peristyle court surrounded by a colonnade of small graceful columns carved out of blue-grey Aphrodisias marble. Communicating with the court to the east, beyond the columns, a triconch or cluster of three apses suggest an official function for this complex of buildings. This is because such a feature in late Roman and early Byzantine residences usually belongs to the palace of a governor or senior official of the state or the church. Its purpose was clearly that of an audience chamber.

date opened into the south portico of the court. In front of them, two smaller, double, blue marble columns had been set up. A well at the side of one of these columns yielded dozens of amphorae, in addition to several glass perfume bottles and their fragments.

Off the western portico, two additional rooms were decorated with multi-coloured, geometrically patterned mosaic floors of the fourth or fifth century. A lateral hall on a higher level than the peristyle court, and with an eastern apsidal end parallel to the triconch, communicated with the court by means of two doors. It contained the remains of a handsome opus sectile floor near its apse. Three more rooms to the south, behind the apsidal ones, seemed to have been topped by an upper storey. The walls showed traces of fresco painting, which had been concealed by coats of rough plaster. When these were removed, two fragmentary but still attractive painted panels were revealed. One of them showed the legs of a characteristic grouping of the Three Graces in a flowering meadow. The second displayed the flimsily draped but headless body of a lovely Nike standing on a globe, her dark wings spread out behind her, her missing arms raised, probably proffering a wreath or an olive branch.

A small bathroom, together with its hypocaust arrangement, and a latrine were uncovered to the side of the southernmost apse of the triconch, to the east of the three south rooms. These features confirmed that the complex had been a private dwelling built in the

Roman times. The obviously pagan nature of the fresco decoration undoubtedly offended the Christian sensibilities of the later inhabitants of the rooms, and it would have been they who daubed them over with plaster.

The size of the triconch unit, the peristyle court and lateral apsidal hall suggested an opulence that in turn suggests some official connection for the complex. Triapsidal, and apsidal, arrangements are often connected with residences of high officials or governors, and referred to as a triclinium unit.

Examples of such formalized dining or reception areas have been found in similar 'palaces' in Libya at Apollonia, at Ptolemais, and at other north African sites. It is therefore reasonable to suggest that the original structure of the Aphrodisias complex was the private residence, or palace, of a late Roman high official, senator, or governor. Its location in a prestigious quarter of the city and its rich decoration provide evidence of the importance of its original owner or occupant. However, the numerous Byzantine remodellings and the discovery of at least one lead seal referring to the 'Metropolitan Bishop of Caria' in the peristyle, may mean that a high Church official subsequently occupied the residence. The proximity of Aphrodisias' main church or cathedral to the north-east would also support such a theory.

Another residential complex with a similarly combined history of Roman and Byzantine occupation was investigated to the north of the temenos of Aphrodite in 1965 and 1966. The building in question, the original construction of which must be assigned a date in the third century, was essentially private in character, but its main unit was a large marble-paved courtyard with an apsidal ending to the west, of impressive dimensions and similar to a triclinium. Beyond the eastern access door was a courtyard. This contained at its centre an attractive, shallow, square pool with moulded edges. The courtyard also included slender blue-grey marble columns and was decorated with a geometric and figurative mosiac pavements, which were, unfortunately, badly damaged. A second, smaller dependency or court with four columns of similar size was excavated south of the triclinium, together with adjoining rooms found alongside and to the north. The numerous finds recorded in this complex indicate a series of occupations and transformations continuing well into the eighth and ninth centuries.

Some aspects of the plan of the residence, particularly the triclinium unit, were reminiscent of complexes found in Athens that related to the teaching of philosophy. In view of the philosophical teaching activities in the second and third centuries associated with the Aristotelian Alexander of Aphrodisias (and, indeed, in the late fifth century with the Neo-Platonist Asklepiodotos), it is tempting to see the original purpose of the building as a school of philosophy which was used after the sixth century for different purposes, including habitation.

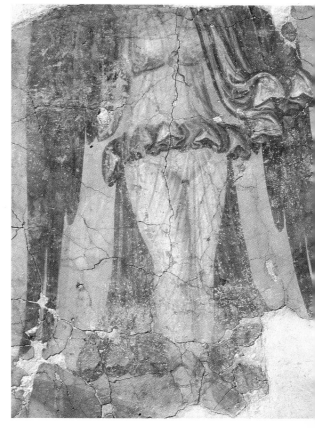

This detail of a fresco painting decorating the wall of one side chamber of the so-called bishop's palace shows a flimsily clad figure of a Nike standing on a globe; it was discovered under a thick layer of plaster. Possibly it belonged to the pagan past of the building and its revealing dress offended the Christian sensibilities of a subsequent occupant.

The 'Acropolis' and Prehistory

The most ambitious and large-scale project undertaken by us at Aphrodisias is undoubtedly the thorough and extensive excavation that focuses on the 'Acropolis' hill. Generously supported by the National Geographic Society, these activities not only yielded highly significant evidence of the prehistory and history of the site, but also brought to light one of its most impressive monuments, the Aphrodisias Theatre.

Early excavators of Aphrodisias had, like Gaudin, labelled the conical hill at the central eastern sector of the ancient city 'Acropolis' — an easy assumption, because it dominated the surrounding neighbouring countryside and suited the role of a citadel remarkably well. Yet its actual origins were neither questioned nor investigated. Surface remains of a large theatre were noted by Gaudin in his brief reports as being visible among the stables and cottages of the east slope, but no effort was made to explore them.

As work continued on the Theatre, the Tetrastoon and the Theatre Baths between 1966 and 1974, investigations were also conducted into the past of the 'Acropolis' - visible behind the workmen on the right of the photograph.

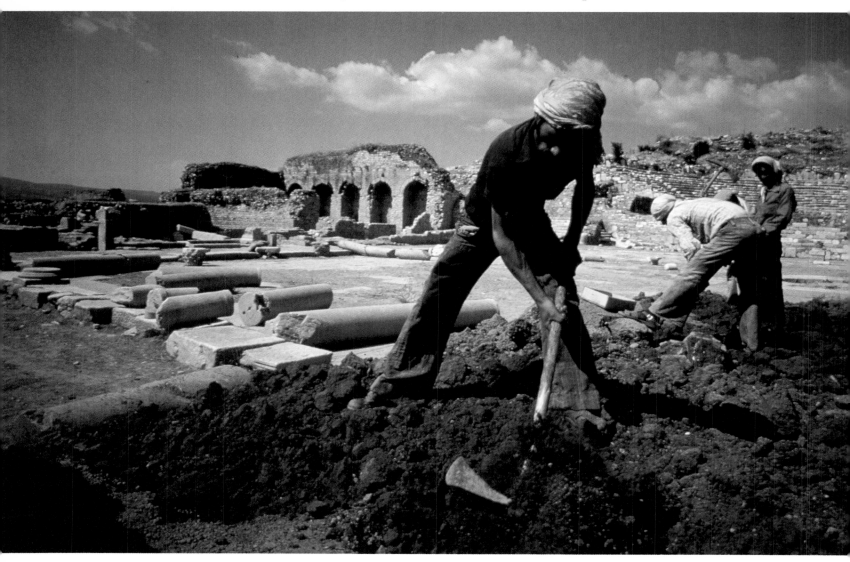

From the beginning of our work at Aphrodisias, however, the regular, conical shape of the 'Acropolis' intrigued us, as it strongly suggested the possibility of some other origin. It was too far from the slopes of Baba Dağ to be the isolated remains of a mountain spur. Nor was it likely to have been purposefully and artificially created to back the construction of the Theatre, or to conceal a burial. The occasional discovery of stone tool fragments in its vicinity and elsewhere in our early investigations strengthened the possibility that the hill was an accumulation of a series of prehistoric settlements — that, in other words the 'Acropolis' was a *höyük*, or artificial habitation mound, equivalent to the near-eastern *tell*. This was substantiated by exploratory probes at the south-western base of the hill in 1966, which yielded obsidian flakes and parallel-sided blades, as well as sherds characteristic of the Anatolian Early Bronze Age (third millenium BC).

About the same time, in 1965 and 1966, probes were undertaken to examine the remains of the Theatre lying between the half-

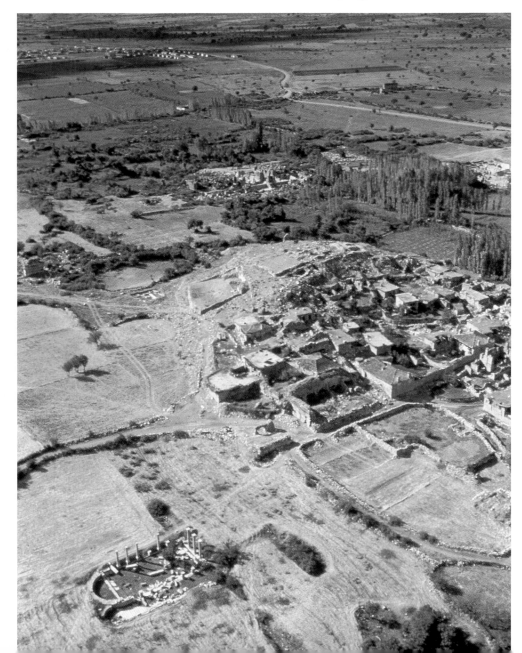

The hillock called the 'Acropolis' is essentially the only elevation in the generally flat site of Aphrodisias. Despite its conventional appellation, this mound is actually a *höyük*, the Turkish equivalent of the Arabic *tell*. This is a prehistoric habitation mound created by successive levels of occupation in which dwellings were made of sun-dried mud bricks. The eastern flank of the 'Acropolis' was dug out for the construction of a large theatre in the first century BC. This theatre was almost completely concealed from view by a number of houses of the village of old Geyre that climbed as far as the top of the hill, inadvertently continuing the ancient habitation pattern. The photograph, taken from the south-east shows this situation prior to excavation of the Theatre, which began in 1966.

The excavated Theatre in the right foreground can be seen cutting into the eastern flank of the 'Acropolis'. The series of deep trenches that were cut into the western half of the 'Acropolis' revealed the prehistoric sequences of habitation of the mound. Fortunately, this portion of the hill was essentially free from later monumental structures. The photograph looks north and shows the 'Acropolis' in relation to other monuments of the site. In a clockwise direction these include the large basilica at the south-western edge of the Portico of Tiberius of the Agora; the Baths of Hadrian on the left of the photograph; the so-called bishop's palace and the Odeon; the poplar groves covering part of the Agora; the remaining houses of old Geyre that concealed the as yet undiscovered Sebasteion; beyond them the Museum; and finally the Tetrastoon and Theatre Baths in front of the Theatre itself.

abandoned houses covering the east slope of the 'Acropolis'. In one of these, at a depth of over seven metres, the stage building was discovered in excellent condition. Such encouraging results spurred a large scale investigation and excavation of the hill and the Theatre on the east slope, as well as the prehistoric settlements on the west side of the 'Acropolis', which was essentially free of Roman or subsequent structures of any significance.

An exhaustive topographical survey of the hill itself and especially its eastern side was completed in 1966, and measures to expropriate the properties involved were set in motion. Eventually all of the half-abandoned or dilapidated cottages were acquired and demolished. Work on the project was initiated the following year and actively continued until 1976. Tons of earth were transported by lorry as far away as possible from Geyre and spread over existing fields, where they proved to be a potent fertilizer. Furthermore, in the case of the Theatre, thousands of architectural blocks and fragments, pertaining to the stage building and other damaged portions, were duly numbered, recorded, drawn and stored in suitable areas nearby, to permit eventual closer scrutiny and study.

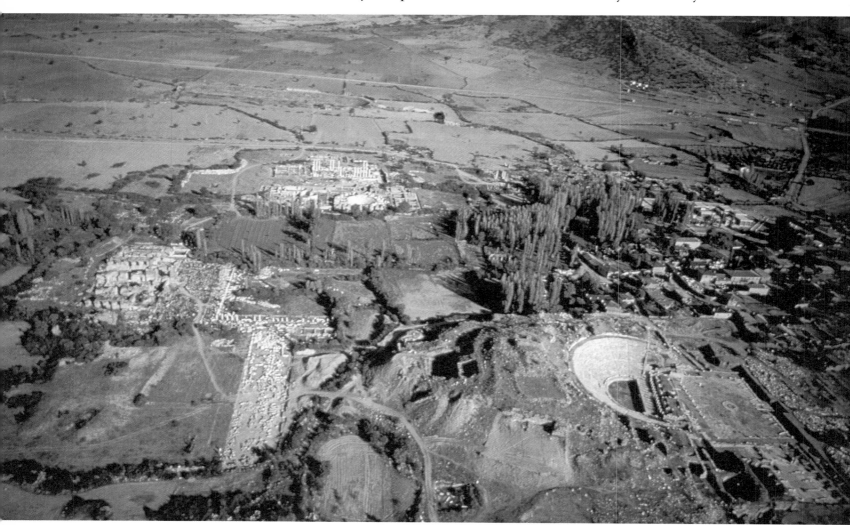

Our investigations into the remote past of Aphrodisias concentrated on the west slope of the 'Acropolis'. Simultaneously, however, sporadic soundings were also conducted in the second mound of the site, located to the east of the 'Acropolis' and referred to as 'Pekmez'.

The carefully organized excavations, and the minute analysis of the results undertaken by Dr. Martha S. Joukowsky, revealed that the prehistory of Aphrodisias antedates its classical past by more than 5,000 years. Its remains dated back to about 5,800 BC, which makes it one of the earliest settlements in Anatolia. Indeed, radio-carbon analysis indicated that the origins of prehistoric life at the site were among the earliest in the Near East. After these first detectable traces of prehistoric habitation, there seemed to have been a hiatus of about 1,500 years. Then, in approximately 4,300 BC, a prominent prehistoric settlement emerged. Evidence indicates that it continued more or less uninterruptedly throughout the Bronze Age and into the Iron Age.

Because of the continuity of successive settlements, Aphrodisias can provide key information for our understanding of prehistoric

A series of painstakingly excavated trenches *(below left)* in the west slope of the 'Acropolis' revealed the extraordinarily rich prehistoric past of the site. Because of the different nature of the archaeological evidence and artefacts connected with this phase of the project, appropriately careful methods, techniques and planning were required for the recovery of evidence. The digging of trenches was often organized in a series of steps and terraces to permit as wide and thorough an analysis as was possible, although eventually the huge depths reached meant that work had to be restricted to the section of one trench only. Early Bronze age artefacts *(below)*, recovered from a *pithos* or large storage jar burial, include a small perfume or unguent bottle, a necklace of thin gold beads, and two silver bracelets.

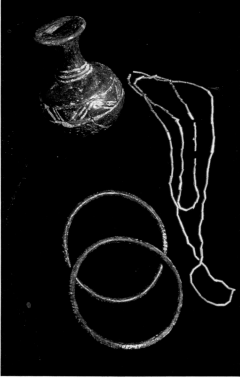

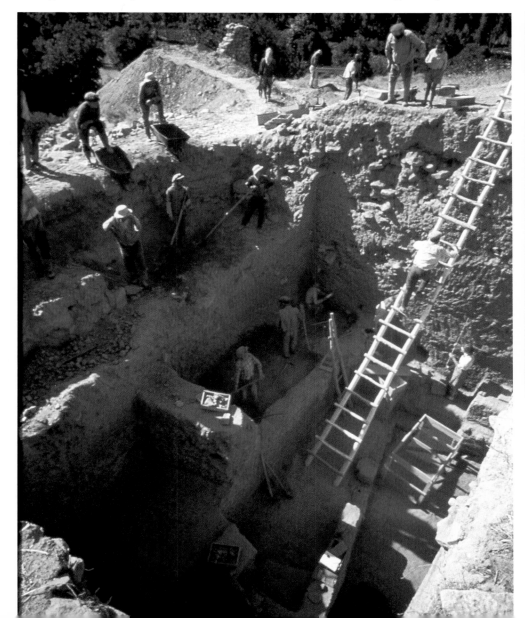

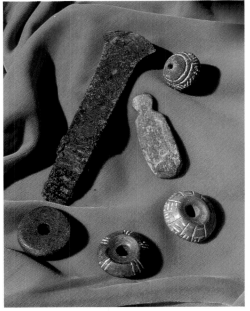

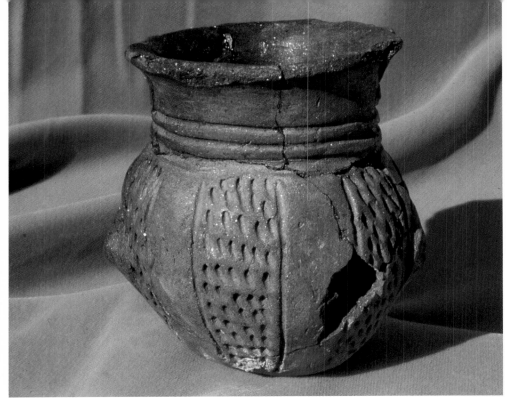

A collection of several typical Bronze Age artefacts recorded from the excavation of the west 'Acropolis' include a small bronze ceremonial axe head, a small stone 'idol', and four spindle whorls. A small handmade early Bronze Age ceramic jar decorated with incised lines and indentations, was among pottery recovered *(above right)*.

developments particular to the south-west of Anatolia. Apart from its contribution to our knowledge of early urban societies in general — their settlement patterns, architectural traits, range of crops and faunal life — the corpus of artefacts testifies to the achievements of the early inhabitants. Among these artefacts, for instance, are figurines that can be dated to the fifth millenium BC, which showed advanced skills of conception and carving. Early technological skills were evidently highly developed. These included working in ground and polished stone, metal and bone; making jewellery in gold and silver; and the production of ceramics. Furthermore, neutron activation tests of obsidian-chipped stone show that Aphrodisias appears to have had contacts with sources of obsidian hundreds of kilometres away — from the Aegean islands to the west, and from central Anatolia to the east — as early as 4,000 BC.

From about 3,000 BC and the early Bronze Age onward, prehistoric Aphrodisias showed close associations or parallels with the important north-western Anatolian site of Troy. Megaroid architecture characteristic of the Aegean and western Anatolia, including Troy, appears among recorded remains; and the remarkable ceramic industry of the inhabitants included *depas* cups, tankards, beak and cutaway spouted jars, large red wheel-made bowls, and incised spindle whorls.

Although parallel developments with Troy and other sites in Anatolia continued through the Middle Bronze Age until the Late Bronze and Iron Age (1600-700 BC), Aphrodisias also enjoyed a distinguished indigenous and independent culture. The cultural and chronological evolution of the site provides us, therefore, with a remarkable continuity of archaeological, anthropological, technological, economic and artistic records of a kind not yet available for any other prehistoric site.

The Aphrodisias Theatre and the Archive Wall

As it stands today, almost entirely revealed, the Aphrodisias Theatre is one of the best preserved and most satisfying monuments of its kind in Turkey. Paradoxically, it was the transformation of the 'Acropolis' into a Byzantine fortress in the seventh century that helped most of all to preserve some of the features of the structure, although it precipitated the damage and destruction of others.

Epigraphic evidence points to a construction date in the second half of the first century BC. The cavea is horseshoe-shaped, like the many Hellenistic theatres of Asia Minor. It was divided into two, perhaps even three diazomata. Unfortunately, the upper parts of this cavea were much damaged in the course of the medieval fortification work, although several upper tiers of seats are still visible in the higher part of the southern side of the hill. Below the preserved diazoma, twenty-seven rows of seats survive in excellent condition. These are divided into eleven cunei and descend to a well-preserved orchestra and stage building. In antiquity the building must have been able to hold close to 8,000 spectators.

Extensive remodelling of the orchestra and adjacent stage building was undertaken in the latter part of the second century. This is confirmed by epigraphic evidence: the main objective apparently being to deepen the pit of the orchestra. In order to achieve this, parts of the stage were modified, and at least two, perhaps even three, of the lowest rows of seats at the level of the orchestra were removed and replaced by a straight supporting high wall. This gave the desired depth to the orchestra and created a conistra arrangement, where popular gladiatorial exhibitions, wrestling bouts and animal hunts or baitings could be accommodated. Additions of wood or iron balustrades before the lowest tiers of seats provided protection for important spectators who were also supplied with decorative marble chairs of honour (proedria) or seated on a special tribunal at the centre of the lower cavea. A small staircase, which could be closed off if necessary, allowed victorious gladiators and athletes to climb up the steps to receive their prizes or palms of honour from the high official presiding over the exhibitions on the tribunal. A water-channel was dug on the floor of the orchestra to bring and evacuate water in order to clean up the excesses of the more brutal activities that took place.

These modifications to the orchestra inevitably had serious effects on the stage building. A number of questions concerning the modifications to which this area was subjected still remain unanswered, but are currently being studied. It is clear however, that the stage itself was widened by the addition of a pulpitum in front of the stage building façade by which it was connected with the cavea. Under this pulpitum, a system of corridors and galleries called the 'via venatorum' was engineered. These were intended for the storage of animals and equipment involved in wild animal hunts and gladi-

Simultaneous with the investigation of the western slope of the 'Acropolis', a major enterprise at Aphrodisias has been the excavation of the large first-century BC Theatre and the later associated Tetrastoon and Theatre Baths. The project was started in 1966 with generous support from the National Geographic Society and, although the excavations have essentially been completed, much remains to be done to restore and protect the monuments and to occasionally extend the exploration of certain sectors. Concurrently the study and preparation for publication of the archaeological evidence is proceeding. As evident on p. 81, the dilapidated houses of old Geyre almost completely hid the remains of the Theatre from view. The burial of the structure is presumed to have been much accelerated by a catastrophic earthquake which occured in the first half of the seventh century AD and caused extensive damage to the whole city. The elaborate stage building and upper tiers of seats of the Theatre completely collapsed into the orchestra pit. Similar wholesale damage has been detected in the Agora, the Odeon and the Sebasteion. The decline of their city, exacerbated by difficult political and economic conditions, prevented the Aphrodisians from ever repairing this damage. Prior to the seventh-century earthquake, a similar disaster had affected the city and in particular disturbed the local water table, but evidently the inhabitants were able to cope with these earlier problems. Threats of invasion and other dangers after the seventh-century earthquake led the Aphrodisians to turn the 'Acropolis' into a fortress by encircling it with fortification walls and building over the ruined Theatre. These activities obliterated most of the upper cavea of the structure which at its apogee could have seated about 8,000 spectators.

atorial exhibitions. One tunnel ran along the whole width of the orchestra and was joined by a perpendicular gallery at the midpoint of the stage. At least one door gave access to the orchestra from the 'via venatorum'. Others appeared to have been blocked at a later date. A series of cuttings on the pulpitum floor imply that here, too, parapets were added for the protection of spectators during some of the exhibitions in the orchestra pit. Other holes and cuttings probably took the supports of stage gear, props or scenery.

It seems possible that the proskenion and the logeion forming the decorative façade (scaenae frons) of the stage building were raised from another position during the second century transformations. Indeed, their attractive arrangement consisting of modified Doric columns, in between which painted panels were inserted in Roman times, should once have been at the level of the orchestra. A similar arrangement can be seen in the charming theatre at Priene. At least one thing suggests that such a modification may have occurred. In its present position the central intercolumniation of the proskenion blocks the finely carved details of the central barrel-vaulted tunnel (porta regia) separating the core of the stage building into two equal halves; had these details originally been invisible to the spectator, such refined carvings would have been unnecessary.

The core of the stage building consisted of six vaulted medium-sized rooms. Four of these had doorways opening on to the corridor space created by the proskenion colonnade, while two communicated with the central barrel-vaulted tunnel. A series of 'label' inscriptions were found cut in the doorways indicating that the rooms were once reserved for storing the accoutrements and equipment of certain popular performers — no doubt the stars of their day. In their front part, these rooms reveal excellent late Hellenistic masonry. Their vaults and back portions, however, were in small-stone technique, probably the result of repairs in the late Roman and early Byzantine period. As with other buildings at Aphrodisias, it is possible that these restorations may have been undertaken after damages caused by one of the earthquakes of the second half of the fourth century.

Most of the Doric half-columns of the proskenion-logeion screening the chambers were found either *in situ* or collapsed in the debris of the fallen upper stage storey. All have been re-erected. Their inscribed architrave blocks have been accounted for and have supplied crucial information concerning the construction date of the Theatre. The inscription proclaimed that the logeion and the proskenion were dedicated "to Aphrodite and to the People (*Demos*)", by G. Iulius Zoilos. Zoilos was described as the "freedman of the son of the divine Julius", that is, of Octavian, who was the adopted son of the deified Julius Caesar. This was the same Zoilos who was inherited as a slave — possibly having been owned by Julius Caesar — and later freed by Octavian, and who subsequently played an important role in the affairs of his native city in the 30s BC. There-

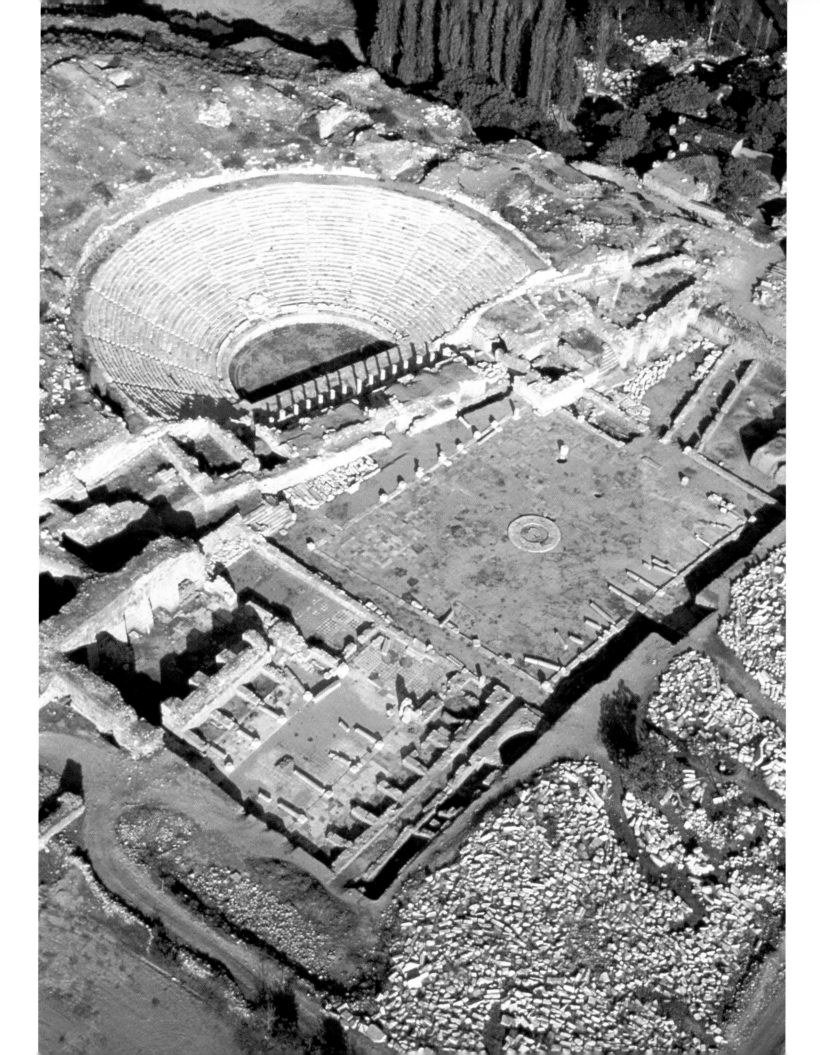

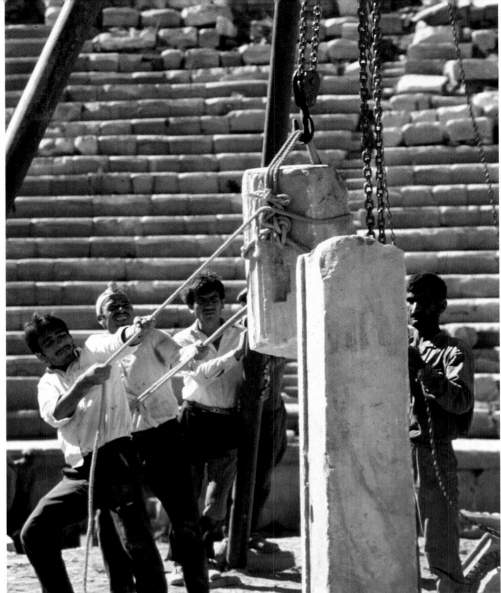

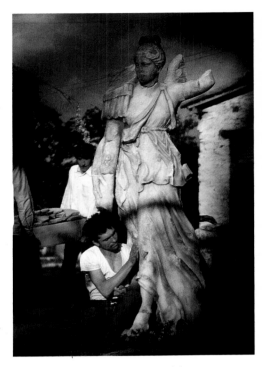

The proskenion and logeion of the stage building complex, now being gradually restored *(above right)*, with all its sculptural decoration, such as the breathtaking Nike figure *(above)*, were originally donated by Gaius Julius Zoilos, a great benefactor of the city and an important figure in the close relationship between Aphrodisias and Rome. The dedicatory inscription *(below and below right)* recording his gift was cut on the architrave block of the proskenion colonnade.

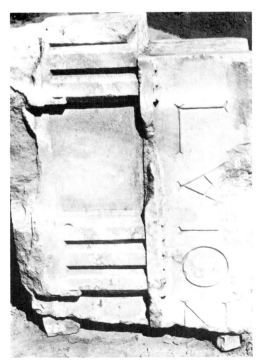

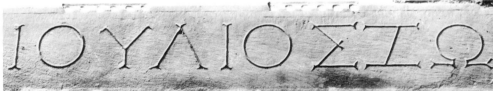

fore the construction of the stage, if not of the whole Theatre, must be dated to this time. It must also be dated before 27 BC, since Octavian's later name, Augustus (or its Greek equivalent, Sebastos), which he adopted at that time, does not appear in the architrave inscription.

Such evidence is of course most significant, not only for the chronology of the Theatre, but also for the dating of the fine decorative elements of the proskenion. During excavations many of these were found trapped in the backstage corridor or fallen on the pulpitum during the collapse of the building. The most exciting among them was unquestionably an elegant, almost baroque statue of a Nike (one of a pair), and several intricately carved floral finial decorations (acroteria).

Even more thrilling was the discovery made in the north parodos, or corridor area, separating the cavea and the stage building itself. As the wall of the building, which was preserved to a height of over five metres and a length of fifteen metres, was being freed from earth and debris, it confronted us with one surprise after another. The whole face of the wall was covered with line after line of well-cut Greek inscriptions. Greek had become the *lingua franca* of much of the eastern Mediterranean after the conquests of Alexander the Great, and continued to be so in Roman times, although Latin was also occasionally used.

It soon became apparent, thanks to the preliminary readings and interpretations of Miss Joyce Reynolds, our epigraphic collaborator, that these documents formed a unique and extraordinarily significant record of the history of Aphrodisias and of Roman Asia Minor. These documents alone could justifiably be referred to as an 'archive'.

In fact, most of the inscriptions were letters. They were cut on the north wall, the south-east corner of the stage building and the adjacent analemma of the north parodos, seemingly in the first half of the third century. They recorded and described events dating from the late Republic and the Second Triumvirate. They also included the *Senatus Consultum de Aphrodisiensibus*, the Roman senatorial decree conferring special status, rank and privileges on Aphrodisias, as well as letters emanating from the emperors Trajan, Hadrian, Commodus, Septimius Severus, Caracalla, Severus Alexander and Gordian III. Regrettably, it is apparent that some fragments of these had been removed from their original position and reused in the city walls.

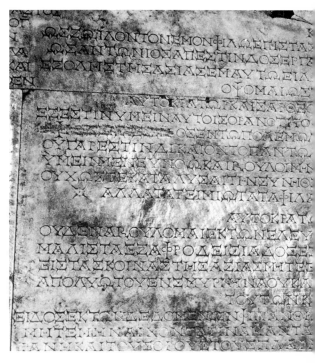

The Aphrodisias Theatre underwent major modifications in the later half of the second century AD to permit certain performances such as gladiatorial games and animal shows to be held in its orchestra. Both at this time and later, the Aphrodisians inscribed on the northern wall of the stage building *(below)* an elaborate series of documents such as the letter from Octavian, at the top of this photograph *(above)*, and other later Imperial communications.

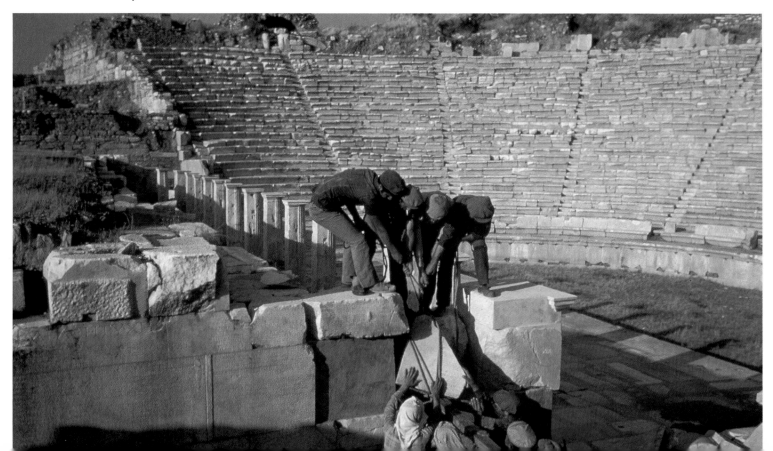

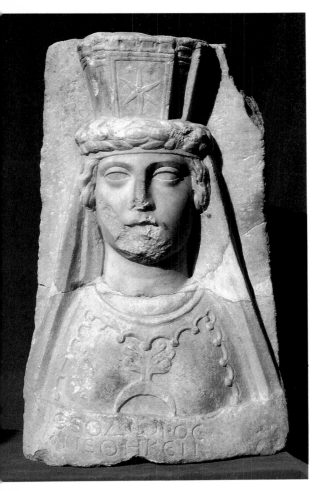

Miraculously saved from damage at Christian hands, this relief bust of the Aphrodite of Aphrodisias, dedicated by a certain Theodoros in the second century AD, adorned the stage façade of the Theatre, from where she looked down serenely upon the audience.

Not unexpectedly, a considerable quantity of sculpture and architectural fragments were discovered on the pulpitum as well as among the debris filling the corridor behind the proskenion-logeion colonnade. All of these pieces are currently in the process of being studied and analysed in efforts to visualize the appearance of the stage as it was in the second and third centuries when Aphrodisias was at its most prosperous. Much of the sculpture has already been restored and is currently exhibited in the Museum. The most interesting piece is an almost intact relief bust of the Aphrodite of Aphrodisias inscribed with the name of its donor, a certain Theodoros. There is also a colossal statue of a handsome young man, with a virtually undamaged, laureate head. According to the inscribed base found nearby, he is symbolic of the *Demos* or people of Aphrodisias.

There was also an unusual trio consisting of two Melpomenes (Muses of Tragedy) framing a draped, headless figure. This figure could have been a tragic poet or maybe even Dionysus or Apollo, both of whom are associated with the theatre and the arts. This group must have been used to adorn the niches of the stage façade. It may be assumed that this was also the function of several other full-length portrait statues that have been discovered in this area. One of them is one of the emperor Domitian, according to its inscribed base; and there is also an exceptionally beautiful statue of an athlete in the style of the fifth-century BC Peloponnesian master sculptor, Polykleitos. Its well-preserved head still bears traces of reddish colouring on the hair and eyes, which implies that it was once well protected in a recess of the Theatre or stage façade.

Two statues of boxers, or pugilists, were discovered in fragments at the north and south edges of the pulpitum and in the orchestra pit. They were probably set up near their respective parodoi's entrance, and reflected the combats that were staged in the orchestra in the late second and third century. They were portraits of two professional athletes, as their faces and bodies betray the characteristic features of their activities: swollen 'cauliflower' ears, broken noses, scar marks, shaven heads with a 'pony-tail' tuft of hair on top, and short, stocky, over-muscular, abused bodies.

The theatre continued in use through the early Byzantine period, but it can be assumed that the more violent types of performance were prohibited or at least scaled down. Damage wrought by the fourth-century earthquakes was repaired. Cubicle or 'chapel' arrangements were created at both ends of the stage corridor of the proskenion-logeion, with bench-like features supported by brick piers, and frescoes on adjacent walls.

Some fragments found in the northern 'chapel' and now reassembled reveal a large-eyed, haloed, male head. An inscription and pieces showing wings identify the figure as the archangel Michael. Stylistically the fresco must be dated to the sixth century. It is a rare example of painted art from this period in the Byzantine world,

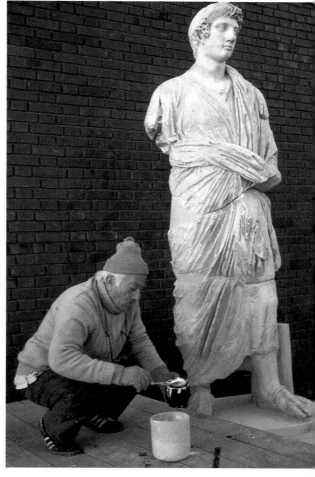

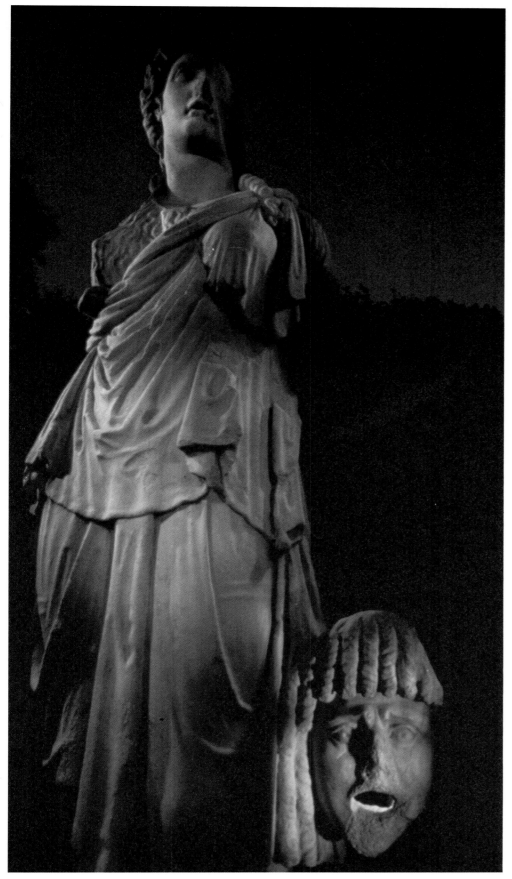

The stage façade of the Theatre was decorated by handsome sculpture. Two of the most stunning examples include *(left)* a first-century AD figure of Melpomene, the muse of tragedy (one of a pair of sculptures), and a handsome youthful depiction from the later first century AD of the *Demos*, or People, of the city, shown above in the process of being restored.

A prized statue that decorated one of the upper niches of the stage building was a beautiful interpretation of the figure of an athlete, the so-called Diskophoros, by a skilled second-century AD Aphrodisian sculptor after the original by the famous fifth-century BC Peloponnesian artist Polykleitos.

The statues of a pair of professional pugilists of the early third century AD, were added to the decoration of the stage when the Theatre underwent modification to allow more violent entertainments to be held in its orchestra area. The overmuscled and battered bodies delineated so remarkably by the sculptor betray the professional and brutal activities of the athletes. The more complete figure is signed on its base by Polyneikes, also known from a signature found in Rome.

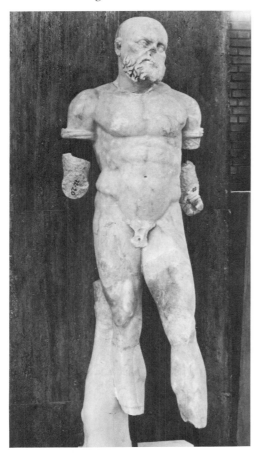

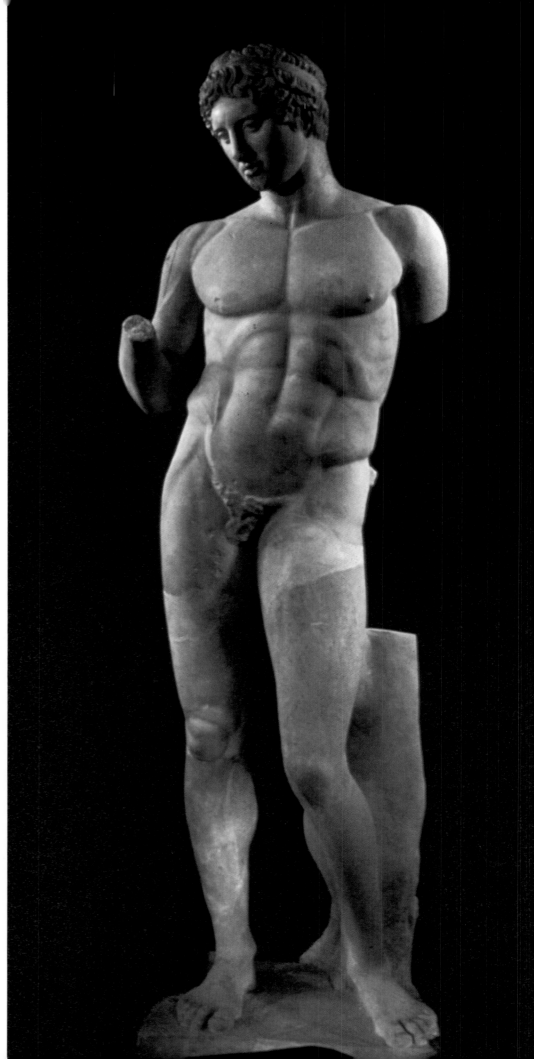

since most early images, icons, mosaics and paintings were destroyed during the subsequent Iconoclastic period.

Additional fragments of contemporary painting were found on the face of the blocked intercolumniations of the proskenion, where painted panels had been inserted in Roman times. Only the lower portions of these decorations have been preserved. Some show plain geometric motifs; others the legs and lower bodies of colourful figures in active postures, perhaps fighting. Numerous graffiti on the seats of the cavea and the walls of the backstage chambers are connected with the later phases of the history of the Theatre. Several mention the "Greens" and the "Blues" — that is, circus "factions", or clubs, no doubt similar to, if not the same as, the clubs or sporting factions of the same names that were so notorious in Constantinople at that time.

According to present evidence, the collapse of the Theatre, and particularly its multi-storeyed stage building may have occurred as a result of a major earthquake in the seventh century during the reign of Heraclius (610-641). Damage resulting from this catastrophe was extremely serious and can be seen in other important buildings in Aphrodisias. The condition of the city did not permit large-scale restoration. In fact, Aphrodisias never recovered and its citizens seem to have lacked either the energy or the expertise to repair their destroyed monuments.

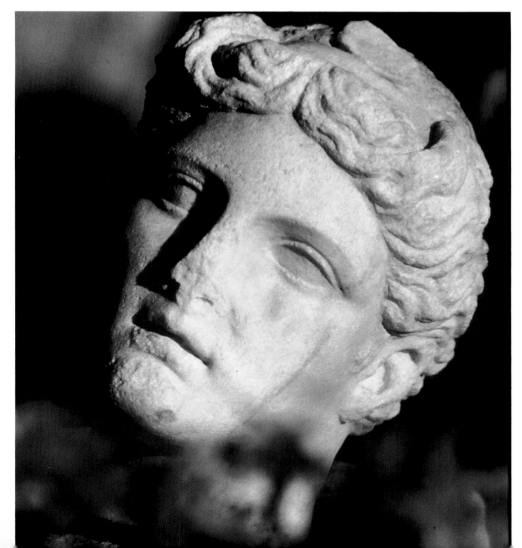

The melancholy countenance of a divine or semi-divine being, found inserted in a wall near the stage building, gazes up wistfully from among flowers.

However, fear of Persian and Arab invaders, or even of brigands, may have forced them to transform the 'Acropolis' hill into a citadel shortly thereafter. The full length of the back of the stage building was blocked by a wall utilizing architectural, epigraphical and sculptural fragments pilfered from neighbouring buildings, including the Sebasteion and the Theatre Baths. In its northward extension, this wall jutted out at a right angle and then resumed a westward direction after another right angle, thus creating a kind of tower or bastion. Beyond this it incorporated a massive earlier buttressed wall, before turning westward along the northern slope of the 'Acropolis'.

This wall can be traced in its major portions, and is seen to have encompassed the whole of the hillock. Several watch-towers were organized along the wall as well as inside the fortress. The ruined remains of the collapsed stage building were not reused, nor were they preserved. What was left of the structure was further destroyed at a later date. The orchestra was filled with dumped material and debris to enable makeshift dwellings to be built both there and on the seats of the adjacent cavea.

From the seventh century on, this citadel must have acted as a refuge. Decimated by plagues and wars, the dwindling population of the city was no longer able to man the three and a half kilometres of fortification walls, although it is possible that the 'Acropolis' walls and other minor buildings could be maintained during relatively peaceful intervals. Yet the destruction of the Theatre, the population's inability to restore it and the need to convert the 'Acropolis' into a fortress left the Aphrodisians without an adequate space for public meetings and entertainment. It was perhaps to fill this need that the large stadium was adapted at its east end to form a structure resembling an arena, with protective cubicles and walls.

The Tetrastoon and Theatre Baths

The original layout in the second and third centuries of the extensive area east of the Theatre, behind and beyond the stage building, is unknown. Excavations conducted here have brought to light subsequent developments, however, and these can be dated to the later fourth century. A large well-paved area, open and approximately square, formed the core of the later layout. A stylobate ran on its four sides, forming porticoes framed by columns on high bases. Several of these were found *in situ* or fallen nearby, although a number were apparently incorporated into the seventh-century stage-blocking wall of the citadel.

Discovery of an inscribed, round, statue base reused in this wall provided a date, as well as a name for this piazza-like arrangement. The base in question mentions the Emperor Julian (the Apostate, 355-365), whose name was subsequently erased and replaced with

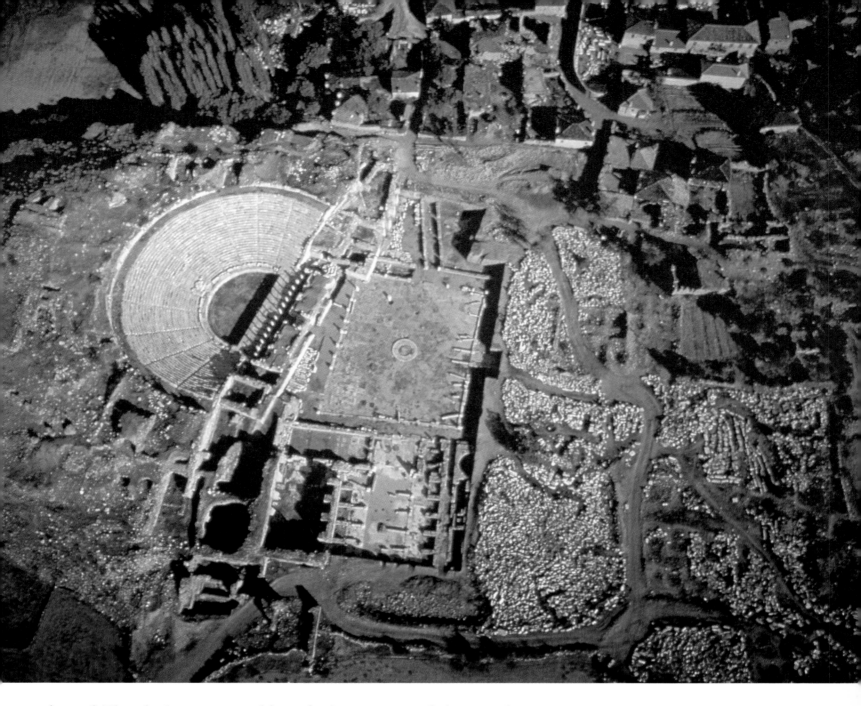

that of Theodosius, presumably referring to one of the two later emperors of that name. The dedicator of the base was a governor of Caria named Antonius Tatianus who, according to the text, built "all the work of the Tetrastoon from its foundations up." There can be little doubt that the word Tetrastoon (four-porticoed area) referred to the piazza-like complex.

The eastern side of the Tetrastoon featured columns resting on normal, rather than high, bases. Several of these were discovered in place but, like other columns of the porticoes, they were not of a uniform type or style, although all were Corinthian. It is safe to assume that they must have been plundered from another building or nearby location. The stylobate of this eastern side also proved to be interrupted at roughly the middle of the portico for a width of about five metres. A sounding to the east brought to light a series of

Following the fourth-century AD earthquakes that resulted in the flooding of the Agora, an area for similar public and market activities was created on higher and drier ground to the east of the stage building. This piazza took the form of a large paved area featuring a circular foundation at its centre and porticoes on each of its four sides - hence its name Tetrastoon. To the south of this piazza can be seen the partially excavated Theatre Baths, originally built in the course of the late second or early third centuries AD.

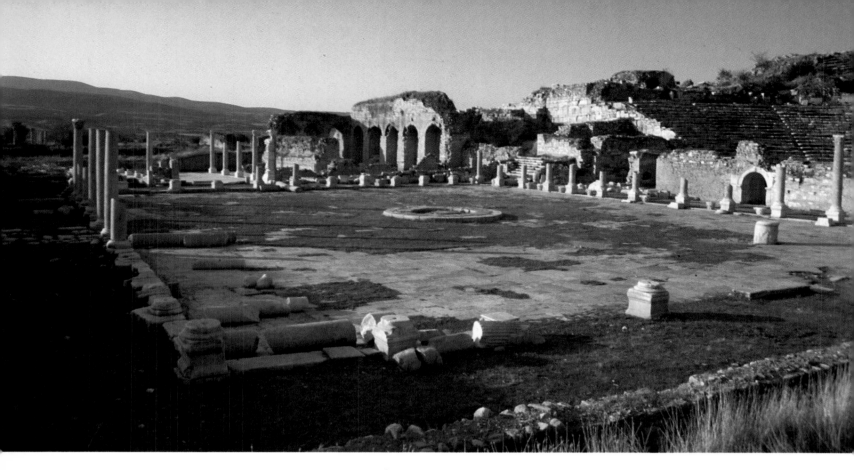

As a public area, the Tetrastoon (*above*) featured several portrait statues of important officials. The arresting portrait of Flavius Palmatus (*below*) was found in front of the portico near the Theatre.

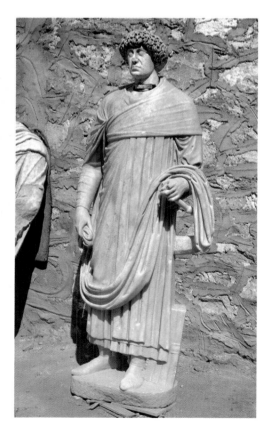

well-cut slabs, the size and surface of which suggest a street or roadway leading to, or coming from, the east.

A circular base or platform was discovered at the approximate centre of the Tetrastoon. It had a diameter of about six metres and included an upright terracotta pipe at its centre, suggesting a fountain-like arrangement. A large, round altar was also found deeply embedded in the regular pavement of the square to the north-east. The body of this altar, once decorated with pagan motifs including garlands and unidentifiable figures, was completely hammered away. Its top surface, however, was cut with lines and barely legible letters, which indicated that the altar had been modified to serve as a sundial.

Two fallen statues were discovered in front of the west portico. Obviously they had originally stood before the colonnade, and had miraculously escaped incorporation within the later stage-blocking of the citadel. One was found near its inscribed base, which identified the statue as the full length portrait of Flavius Palmatus, a 'vicar' (or governor) of the administative district of Asiana. Palmatus is shown in full toga with a broad contabulatio. In his right hand he grasps the *mappa*, or handkerchief insignia of his rank, which was used to signal the opening of festivals or games; in his left hand he holds his sceptre of office. The character of his strong-featured portrait-head makes it a remarkable specimen of the art of fifth-century Aphrodisian sculpture when classical marble-carving traditions were on the wane.

To the south of Palmatus, a much earlier, first-century sculpture was recovered: this was a sensitively modelled, draped body of a

90

young boy, also in full toga. An excellent portrait head that was found nearby almost certainly belonged to it. The face is that of a melancholy youth, wearing an elaborate diadem consisting of separately inserted cameo-like elements, sadly now lost. Upon careful examination, the portrait head was revealed to have been skilfully reworked in the fourth century from an earlier head, to show a prince of the Constantinian house, perhaps Constantine II (337-340) or Constantius II (337-362).

Several small probes under the pavement of the square did not produce any clear evidence of whatever existed behind the stage building before the fourth century. It is probable that the building or buildings that were here were seriously damaged by the earthquakes of the mid-fourth century, or shortly thereafter, and their remains were demolished to make way for the Tetrastoon. There can be little doubt that the Tetrastoon acted as a market-area, or agora.

Since Aphrodisias was endowed with a handsome and extensive agora complex stretching between the north flank of the 'Acropolis' and the Odeon, the addition of another similar public place is puzzling. The answer may well be connected, yet again, with the fourth-century earthquakes which, as evidence from other excavations — the Odeon, the Sebasteion and the 'Agora Gate' — has revealed, strongly affected the water table of the area and the canalizations that channelled water into the city. Serious flooding probably followed, and the first-century agora, which is situated in the lower lying area, must have been particularly badly affected. Because of this, another public market-area would have been organised behind the theatre stage on higher and drier ground until the inundations of the original agora could be stemmed.

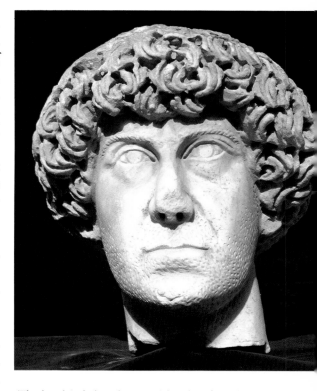

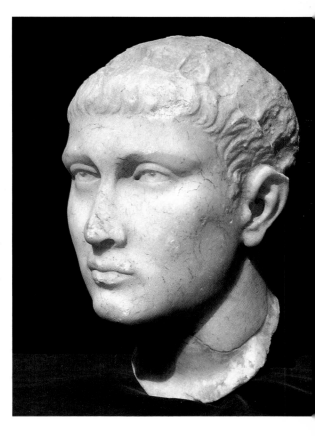

The heads of Fl. Palmatus *(above)* and a prince of the Constantinian dynasty *(below)* exemplify the skills of the Aphrodisian school of portraiture.

The market and shopping areas of the Tetrastoon were not limited to the square area behind the Theatre stage. They appear to have overlapped a complex located to the south, extending beyond the south portico and the adjacent cavea of the Theatre to the west. Identification of this area was again helped by an inscription extracted from the stage-blocking wall. This document, another statue base, honoured a certain Dulcitius, a fifth-century governor of Caria, and was said to have been "set up in front of the baths". These baths could not have been the more distantly located Baths of Hadrian, which were excavated by Gaudin, but must have been another, nearer, thermal establishment.

Sporadic investigations in the complex of ruins south of the Tetrastoon brought to light several halls with a number of terracotta water-pipes inserted into their masonry. One of these, immediately south of the market-place, was thought for a while to have been a fountain-house or 'nymphaeum'.

The most spectacular unit of the complex was a miraculously well-preserved circular room. This was located to the west of the nymphaeum with which it communicated through two slanting vaulted corridors. The features of this room fully affirmed the use of this building as a thermal establishment. The excavators accordingly referred to the complex as the Theatre baths.

The condition of the structure's circular hall was truly remarkable. Its walls stood to a height of over ten metres. Its roof, now collapsed, must surely have been a dome. It featured four main arcuate, apsidal or semi-circular niches opposite one another at the four cardinal points. Two of these niches had smaller, subsidiary doors or passageways, also vaulted. The south-eastern one had three

Because of a village road and unexpropriated property to the south, the continued excavation of the Theatre Baths has had to be delayed. However two of the most extraordinary and well-preserved units of this establishment have been revealed and partially restored. One is a circular domed calidarium arrangement, the walls of which feature apses, once revetted with attractive marble plaques.

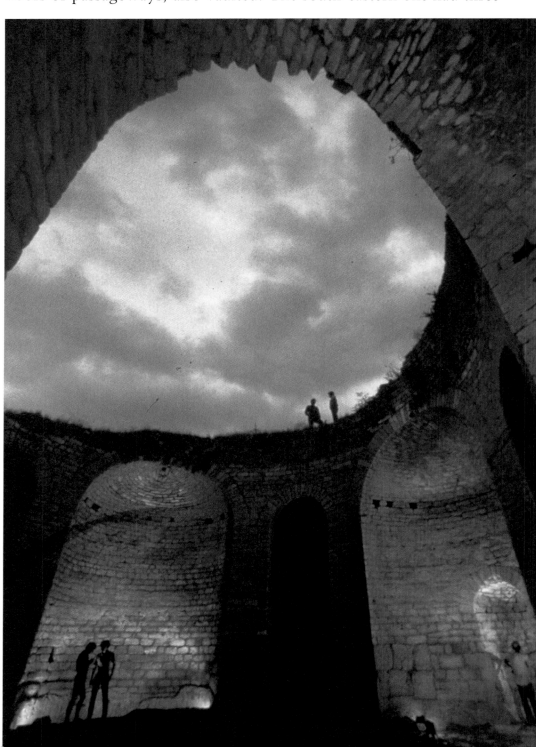

such passages, one of them communicating with the nymphaeum hall, another leading to a hypocaust arrangement partly excavated to the south. The north-eastern niche was also broken by a passage leading to the nymphaeum hall. In addition, four small, subsidiary, arcuate, but almost rectangular recesses came to light between the main niches.

The internal layout of this bathing hall, or *aula termale*, included two contiguous pools, separated by a low wall. The greater part of this arrangement must be attributed to Byzantine modifications, as a Roman architect or designer would not have placed a rectangular internal feature inside a circular structure. The pool to the west was polygonal and shallow; the adjoining one rectangular and deeper, and occupied more than half of the interior of the hall. The presence of a system of upright terracotta pipes and steam-conducting hollow tiles at its eastern end suggests that the *aula termale* was a calidarium or a hot, steam bath unit. The four large main semicircular niches appeared to have been used as shallow receptacles or basins.

Another hall was located to the east of the nymphaeum unit and communicated with it through two side doors. It formed a striking and lavishly decorated element in the plan of the basilica. Oriented north-south, it featured a nave separated from its aisles by Corinthian colonnades made of local blue-grey marble, standing on high bases. In both of its aisles, short curtain walls formed small rooms that were probably used as shops or booths. The pavement of the nave was very well preserved and consisted of closely fitted large marble slabs. The nave seems to have been open to the sky, except at its northern extremity, where two rectangular pillars of blue-grey

The other beautiful discovery is a hall with the plan of a basilica *(below)* featuring very well preserved marble paving and exquisite blue-grey marble Corinthian columns, separating the nave from the aisles. The far end of the 'basilica' hall terminated in a rectangular recessed area that would have appeared framed as one approached it by two beautiful 'peopled scrolls' pillars joined by a similarly decorated arch. It is possible that the statue of an emperor stood within this recess. During the creation of the Tetrastoon, immediately to the north, in the late fourth century AD the statue would have been removed and a door cut through between this hall and the Tetrastoon. The hall thus became a part of the piazza area, and stalls or shops were probably created in its aisles.

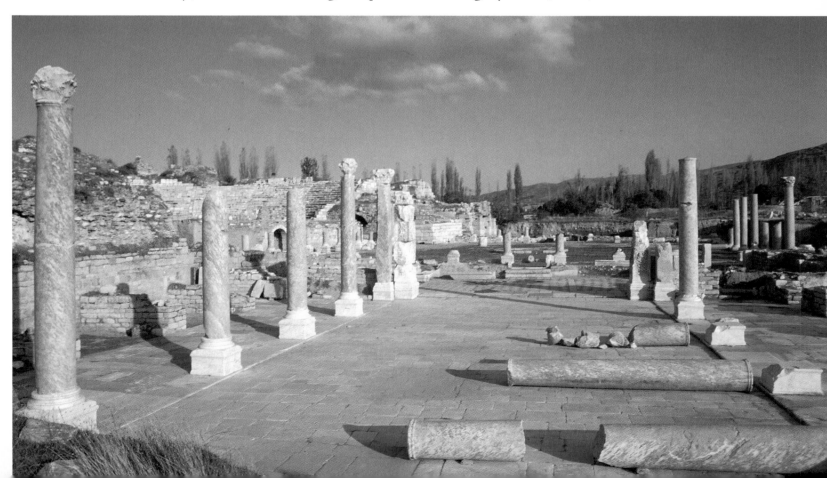

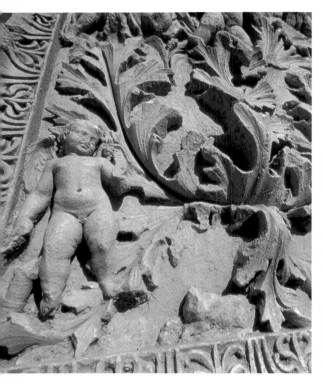

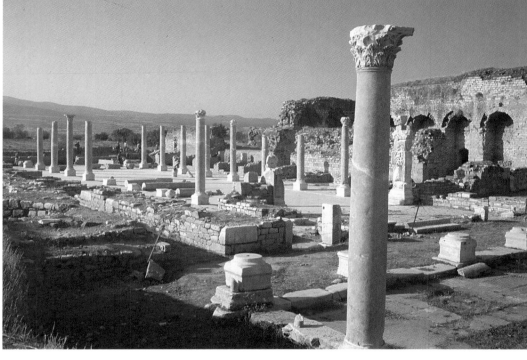

The recessed area of the 'basilica' hall featured typically Aphrodisian 'peopled scrolls' pillars *(above)* portraying endearing figures of Erotes hunting various animals among the luxurious vegetation of acanthus leaves.

The connection between the Tetrastoon and the Theatre Baths can be seen *(above right)* at the north end of the 'basilica' hall, marked by two shallow steps leading from the piazza to the recessed area of the hall.

marble aligned with the aisle colonnades and rested against two pilasters framing a chamber or 'oecus', which formed the northern end of the hall.

Both of these pilasters were intricately carved in the 'peopled scrolls' style much favoured by Aphrodisian sculptors. Similar carvings were also discovered in the decoration of the Baths of Hadrian, excavated by Gaudin in 1904. Lions, stags, birds and Eros-figures jumped, ran, frolicked and flew among elaborately intertwining swirls of acanthus on the south and internal faces of the pilasters. A number of other fragments carved on one face with acanthus scrolls and flowers were found nearby. One of them showed the mask of a Medusa head, another favourite Aphrodisian motif. The imperceptibly curved shape of these blocks suggested that they formed part of an archway joining the two 'peopled scrolls' pilasters, and that the block with the Medusa head was its keystone.

The specific original function of this elegantly decorated recess or chamber remains uncertain. Obviously, the area that the pilasters framed was the focal point of the basilica hall. It is plausible that an important statue (or group of statues) was located in the oecus, which was paved with attractive black and white marble slabs. The statue may have been of an emperor and was probably removed in the fourth century. At that time, a door was cut through the northern wall of the chamber to connect it with the south portico of the Tetrastoon. The basilica hall then became an extension of the Tetrastoon market area and the cubicles formed by the short curtain walls of its aisles would have been used as shops or 'tabernae'.

The passage of a local road leading from old Geyre to vineyards and fields situated to the south, and the presence of large tracts of unexpropriated land near the Theatre Baths prevented continuation of work in this area. Nevertheless, in 1982 and 1983 most of the blue-grey columns framing the nave of the basilica hall were re-erected, along with parts of the 'peopled scrolls' pilasters. These and similar restorations in the Tetrastoon greatly enhanced the already impressive general appearance of the whole area.

The Baths of Hadrian and the Museum

At the beginning of our present series of excavations in 1961 — even before the extraordinary harvest of important finds — our plans for the future of Aphrodisias had included a museum located at the site. Several projects were drawn-up, and suitable places were examined and explored.

For a while, in 1965, the possibility of using an ancient building — specifically, the halls of the Baths of Hadrian — discreetly adapted and restored, was seriously considered. The idea of exhibiting sculpture in a thermal establishment was certainly not new, as such projects had been realized elsewhere. Indeed, in their own time, Roman baths were known to have been repositories for statuary and their halls were filled with many bronze and marble figures.

In order to explore the feasibility of this solution at Aphrodisias, excavation activities were resumed in 1965 in the Baths of Hadrian. Only the entrance-court, or 'palaestra', and part of the Portico of Tiberius adjacent to the Agora, had been investigated by Paul Gaudin. Boulanger, in 1913, and the Italian mission of 1937 had also made limited probes in the north-western corner of this area.

The Baths of Hadrian consisted of an approximately symmetrical grouping of two large galleries on either side of a huge central hall. This hall was probably the calidarium, and featured elaborate underground servicing corridors, barrel-vaulted tunnels, furnace-rooms and water-channels. We were first confronted with the difficult task of removing many large tufa blocks with which the core of the building was built. These had fallen from the upper walls where originally they had been covered, or revetted, with decorative marble plaques.

Following the laborious clearance of the calidarium and its hypocaust arrangement, two of the parallel and contiguous galleries to

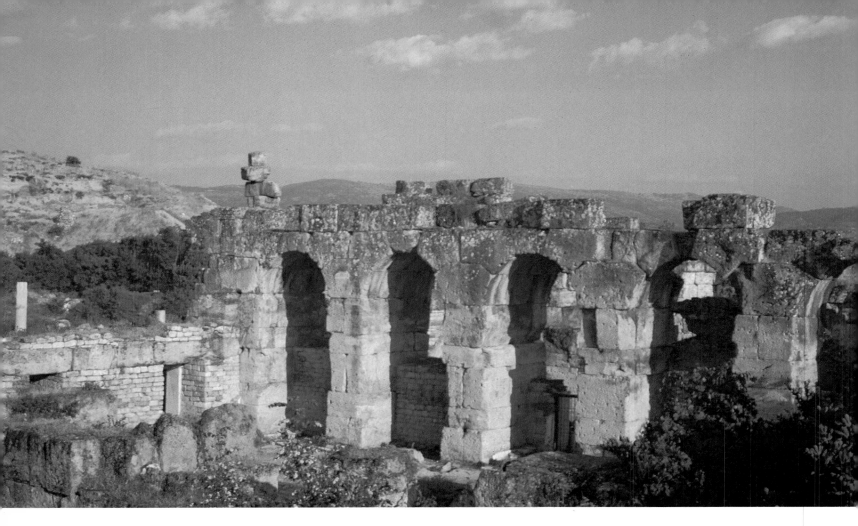

Like many other Anatolian cities in Roman times, Aphrodisias must have boasted several baths apart from the ones located by the Theatre. An even larger establishment than the Theatre Baths, and the site of the earliest excavation at Aphrodisias in 1904-1905, is known as the Baths of Hadrian *(above)*. The building was so-called after the discovery by Gaudin in 1904 of a dedicatory inscription to that emperor. The sudatorium *(opposite above left)* of the Baths of Hadrian included a shallow central pool and marble floor, supported by small terracotta pillars that allowed space for the circulation of heated air beneath the floor from a central furnace.

the north were excavated. The one immediately next to the calidarium was probably a lukewarm room or 'tepidarium', with its own hypocaust system. To the east, it led into a large room that contained a shallow, circular pool, supported by square hypocaust pillars and revetted with marble. It must have served as a sweat room, or 'sudatorium'.

The sudatorium could also be entered through another large chamber to its north, perhaps a dressing-room, or 'apodyterium'. The excavation of this last chamber created great excitement in 1966, for on the threshold of its western door leading to the second gallery, parallel to the tepidarium, were three colossal and superb marble heads recovered along with other handsome debris. One of the heads was an impressive portrait of a second-century noblewoman wearing a diadem, probably the insignia of the priesthood of Aphrodite. The other two were beautifully executed heads of Aphrodite and Apollo. The pupils of the god's eyes still bore traces of paint, while red underpaint and fragments of gilt still adhered to the abundant hair.

Farther north, another gallery was cleared, parallel to the core of the baths and those galleries already found. Its specific function is not certain, but it may well have served as another dressing or undressing hall. Communicating with it to the east, and with the apodyterium to the south, we discovered what may have been a cold room, or 'frigidarium'.

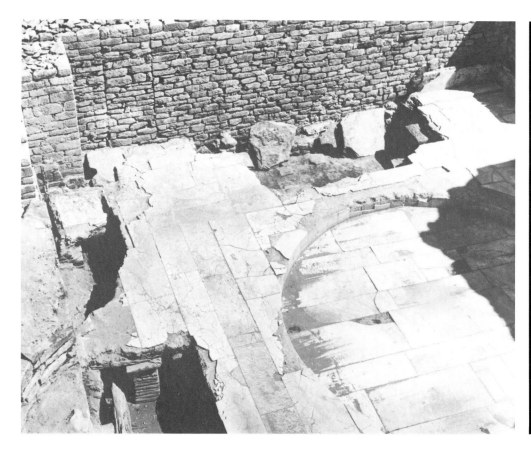

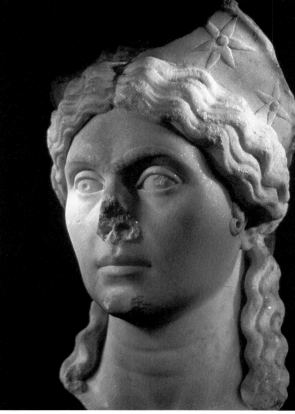

Like all Roman baths, the Baths of Hadrian were lavishly decorated with sculpture. Two beautiful examples include a large second-century female portrait head *(above)* and a superbly rendered head of Apollo *(below)*.

At the centre was a rectangular pool, marked by a massive column at each of its four corners and framed by a moulded balustrade. Several beautifully carved fragments of sculpture were discovered inside and outside the pool. Although battered, one of them, a handsome large nude male torso, and another, the limp body of a draped female figure, were easily identified as the key elements of the well-known Achilles and Penthesilea group of late Hellenistic date. The Greek hero of the Trojan War was shown dragging the body of the Amazon queen Penthesilea, whom he had just killed in single combat. The size of the group made it suitable for one of the two platforms that fitted on either side of the pool.

As excavations proceeded, following the discovery of the two figures of Achilles and Penthesilea, the possible identities of the sculptures occupying the second platform were the subject of much speculation. The most likely answer seemed to be a group representing Menelaus dragging the slain Patroclus, faithful companion of Achilles. To our delight, fragments — although regrettably no more than fragments — of this equally famous late Hellenistic sculpture were recovered, battered but still recognizable, from the interior of the pool.

Although much more information about the Baths was needed and the prospects of finding additional joining fragments for the statuary were tempting, the condition of the area north of the frigidarium, and particularly that of the other large galleries to the south,

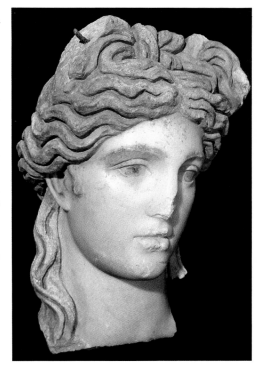

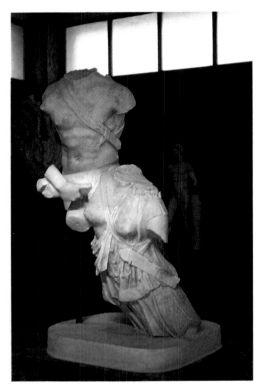

Another notable discovery in the Baths was a partially preserved group showing Achilles dragging the body of the Amazon queen Penthesilea, killed by him in single combat in the Trojan war.

appeared less than satisfactory. Indeed, the friable nature of the tufa of these galleries' upper arches and vaults seemed quite seriously affected by long exposure to the elements and damaged by fire. Furthermore, to complete the project, it would have been essential to expropriate considerably more of the nearby properties. Finally, because the estimated cost of restoring and refurbishing the Baths and transforming the galleries into exhibition halls was so staggering, and in consequence so controversial, excavation of the large complex had to be postponed.

Surface investigations, the search for missing architectural or epigraphical fragments and some restoration activities have continued in the general area of the Baths of Hadrian. More specifically, work has concentrated on the Portico of Tiberius in the nearby Agora.

Following careful study of their component parts, more than eight Ionic columns forming the northern half of the west end of the portico adjacent to the Baths were reassembled and re-erected on their plinths to their full height in the autumn of 1983. In 1970, and then again in 1977, surface exploration of a structure abutting the south colonnade of the Portico of Tiberius, near the baths, proved fruitful. A colossal, yet sensitively executed draped female statue, either an empress or a goddess, was recovered. There was also a

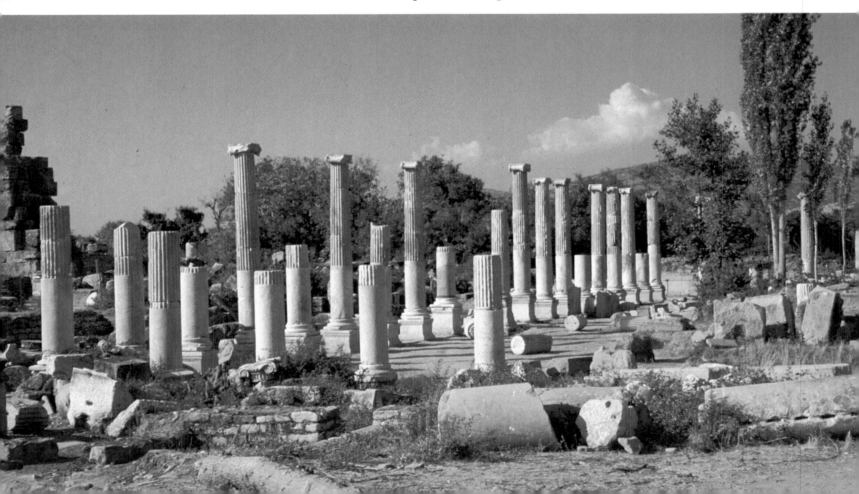

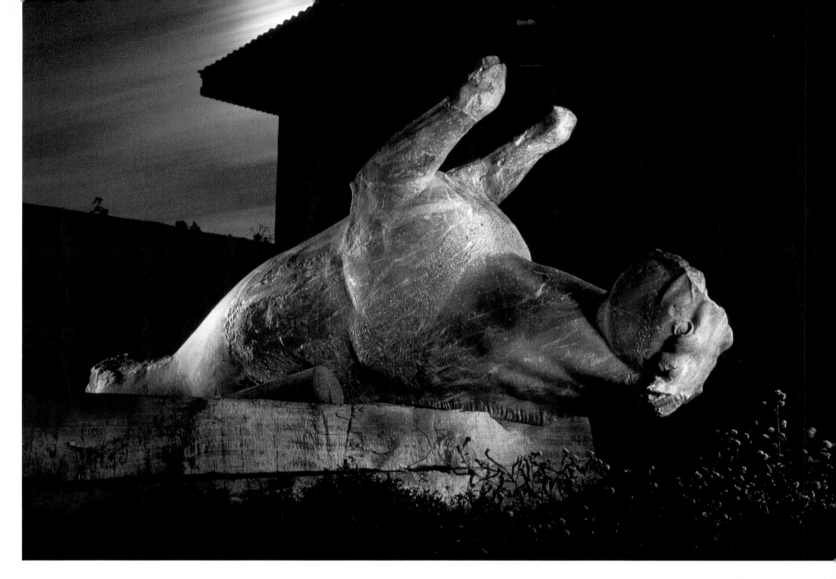

beautiful, though mutilated, lifesize figure of a running horse, carved from blue marble. Unfortunately only fragments of its rider, which had been carved out of dramatically contrasting white marbles, were found.

Many pieces of inscribed panels had been discovered scattered near the surface in this area, both by Jacopi in 1937 and by our own teams. These panels recorded the famous *Edict of Maximum Prices*, promulgated by the Emperor Diocletian in 301. Casual search produced two other large sections of inscribed panels. These proved, however, to belong to a companion decree, heretofore unknown, although its existence had been suspected.

Study of these texts by Miss Joyce Reynolds suggested that the subject matter concerned coinage and that the problems at issue were the payment of public and private debts and the reform of the Roman currency. No archaeological discovery could have been more topical, as the then Prime Minister of Turkey had announced a devaluation of the Turkish currency only a few days before. His words concerning his inflation curbing measures seemed to echo those of Diocletian, 1,600 years before.

The remains of a large structure where Diocletian's decrees appeared to have been exhibited, attracted our attention in 1977. As

An extraordinary and powerfully modelled figure of a running horse *(above)* carved in blue-grey marble is seen here just after its discovery. The horse was unearthed in an uncertain context at the end of the row of columns at approximately the left edge of the photograph opposite. Only the thigh of its rider has been subsequently found. This is in white marble which would have contrasted dramatically with the darker horse in the original equestrian statue. The use of different coloured stones to create a cameo-like effect appears to have been one of the special innovative characteristics of Aphrodisian sculptors.

The Baths of Hadrian communicated directly with the Agora of the city through the west end of the Portico of Tiberius *(opposite)*. This area was briefly investigated in 1904 and has been the scene of continued activity in recent years. A great many of the Ionic columns of the portico have been identified and re-erected.

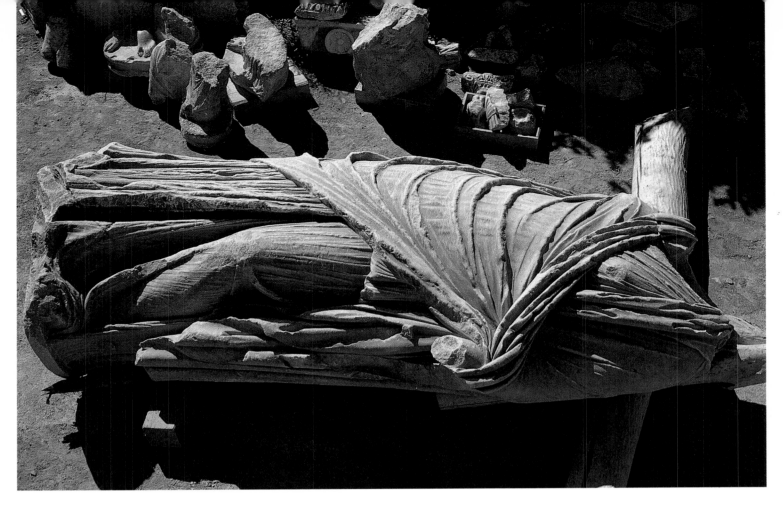

The massive, draped, female standing figure was found near the blue-grey marble horse.

Inscribed panels displayed in front of the large basilica recorded Diocletian's *Edict of Maximum Prices*.

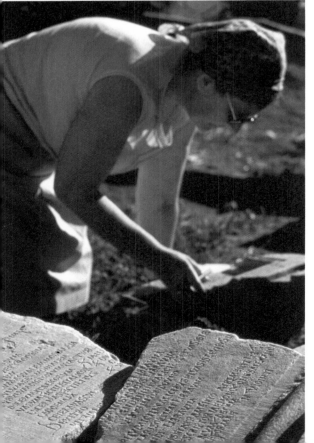

these remains lay close to the surface, a general survey and additional probes were undertaken. These revealed that the building was a substantial large basilica, consisting of a large nave and two aisles, the whole extending southward for a length of over one hundred metres. The size and location suggested a connection with the administrative and legal activities of public life. Its original construction may well have been in the late first century, but evidence indicated that it assumed greater importance in the second half of the third century. It was probably at this time that relief panels forming a balustrade for the upper intercolumniations of the east aisle were added.

Among the figures represented on these reliefs, and duly identified with inscriptions, were Ninos and his wife Semiramis, shown in Roman dress. Also portrayed were Apollo, Pegasus, Bellerophon, and Gordios. The simultaneous presence here of Ninos (mentioned by Stephanus of Byzantium as the founder of Ninoë, alias Aphrodisias) and Gordios, the mythical king of Phrygia, is thought-provoking. It may even be considered to be corroborating evidence of Aphrodisias' importance in the joint province of Caria and Phrygia created in the second part of the third century. The relief panels can be dated to this time on stylistic grounds. The presumed enlargements, additions and decoration of the basilica could also be interpreted as signs of the new significance gained by the building as an administrative and official centre for the capital of the joint province.

100

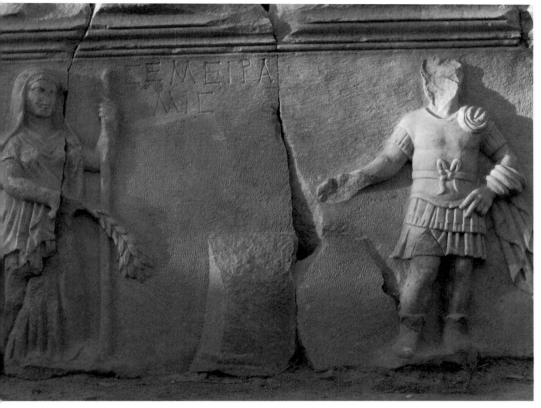

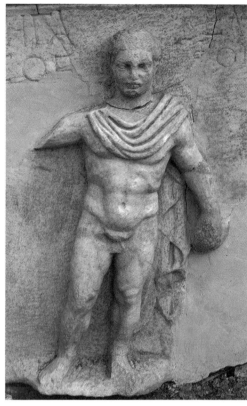

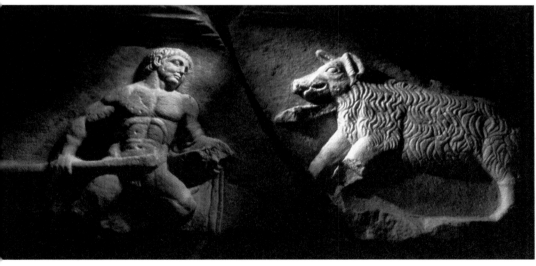

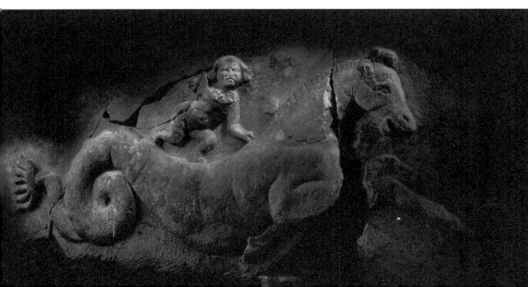

Although its date is as yet uncertain because excavation is incomplete, the original construction of the larger basilica may well have occurred in early Imperial times. It seems clear, however, that the building underwent major adaptation and enlargement in the second half of the third century AD. These activities might be connected with Aphrodisias becoming for a while the capital of a reorganized joint province of Caria and Phrygia. The basilica was a necessary building complex for the provincial and other official business connected with this new administrative role. In this context, a series of balustrade relief panels were probably placed between the columns of the second storey of the aisles of the basilica. These proclaimed the antiquity as well as the mythological connections of Aphrodisias and portrayed figures – some in contemporary garb – that purportedly played a role in the foundation of the city. They include King Ninos, Queen Semiramis performing sacrifices at an altar with Gordius, mythical king of Phrygia *(above left)*; the heroes Bellerophon *(top right)* and Meleager, shown spearing the Calydonian boar *(centre)*, and other subjects such as Eros riding a hippocamp. The panels were also decorated with floral motifs.

After we were forced to abandon the idea of creating a museum at Aphrodisias within the halls of the Baths of Hadrian, the rapidly increasing accumulation of our varied archaeological material, and in particular of large sculptures, made the construction of an appropriate museum building urgently necessary. The old storage depot located in the village square of Geyre, as well as our own facilities, were literally filled to capacity with pottery boxes, sculpture and inscribed fragments of all sizes.

Several sets of plans for a new building were prepared and discussed with the Directorate-General of Antiquities and Museums. A suitable location was selected not far from the old storage depot, and potential donors and contributors were approached. Unfortunately, no positive response was forthcoming. In 1971, however, the Directorate-General took the initiative, following our repeated requests for help, and allocated initial funds for the expropriation of the property selected as a site for the museum. The design of the plans was then entrusted to a government-employed architect.

The following year, the National Geographic Society, a staunch financial supporter of the excavations since 1966, matched the initial funds that had been allocated by the Turkish authorities. Foundations were dug in 1972 and rough concrete construction began later the same year. Progress, which depended on annual Turkish subsidies, proved to be slow. In 1977 and 1978, however, the building was sufficiently far advanced to receive most of the sculpture that was intended to be displayed in its halls. Under our supervision, restoration work on this material was able to be started subsequently.

Prior to the completion of the Aphrodisias Museum in 1971 by the Turkish authorities, restoration activities were undertaken in the storehouse depot *(below)*. The statues of the youthful Herakles and the torso of Aphrodite can be identified.

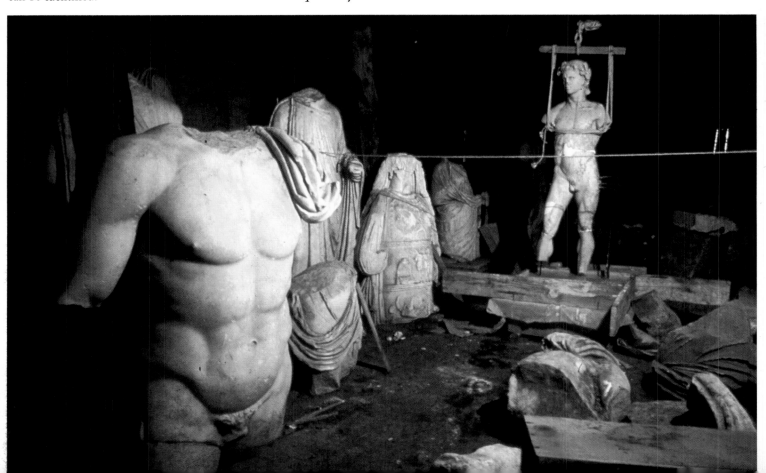

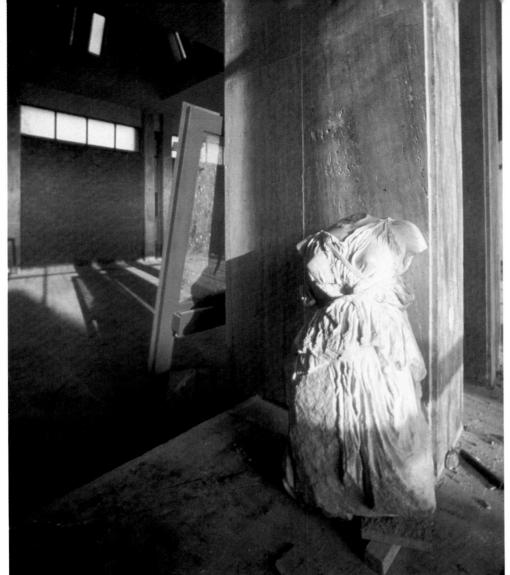

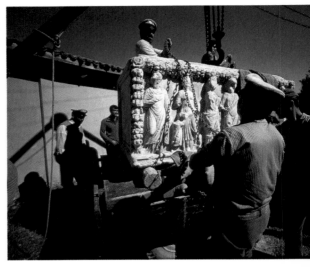

When the Museum building was ready to receive its future occupants, the laborious and careful task of transferring items selected for display began. These included huge sarcophagi *(above)* as well as more delicate statuary and fragments, such as the Artemis torso *(left)* and the Athena head *(below)*.

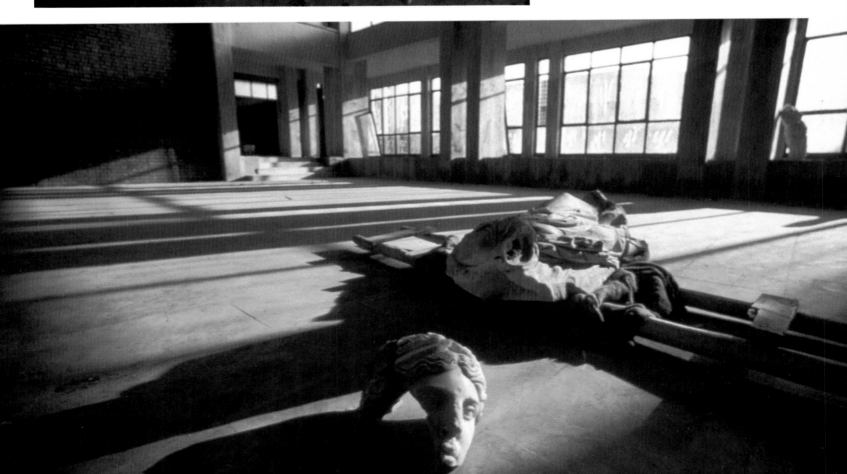

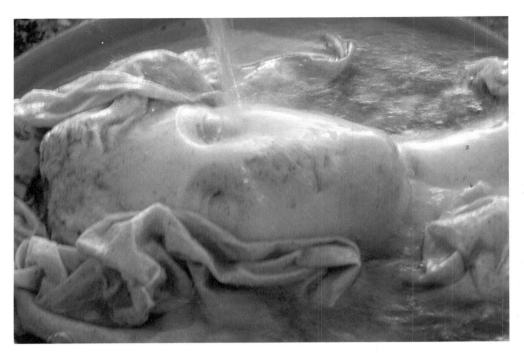

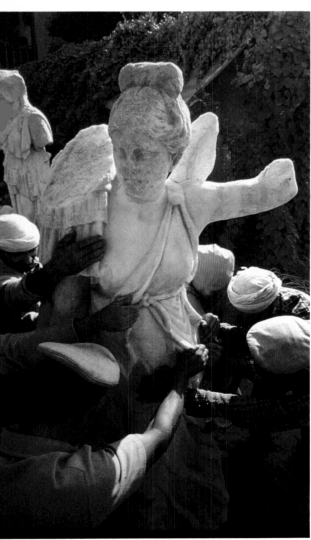

After many frustrating difficulties and delays, the Aphrodisias Museum was officially inaugurated by the Governor of the Province of Aydin, the Honourable Munir Guney, on July 21 1979. Many details were left incomplete and others — perhaps inevitably — proved to be unsatisfactory. Nevertheless, the occasion marked the start of a momentous phase in the history of Aphrodisias and of our association with it.

However important in itself, the completion and inauguration of the museum was nevertheless only one step toward establishing a broader and more urgent perspective regarding the site. The notion of Aphrodisias as a complete archaeological unit, incorporating a museum building as well as an extensive site, or open air museum, needed clear definition. To this end it became vital to safeguard and sanction all things relating to Aphrodisias both within and beyond the perimeter of the ancient city's fortification system.

In 1976 the Turkish High Commission for Monuments (Yuksek Anıtlar Kurulu) approved protection plans for the site which had been prepared in conjunction with the Directorate-General of Antiquities and Museums. Following our frequent and insistent representations, the Directorate-General agreed to accelerate the expropriation of the remaining village houses of Geyre, the condition of which had not changed since the 1960s. By 1979, a great many of these had been acquired and emptied, and several had begun to be dismantled by their former owners.

In the course of these demolitions, many unusual discoveries were made, proving not only that much of the core of ancient Aphrodisias lay under the former houses of Geyre, but also that some of the most significant structures were located in the central eastern sector of the ancient city.

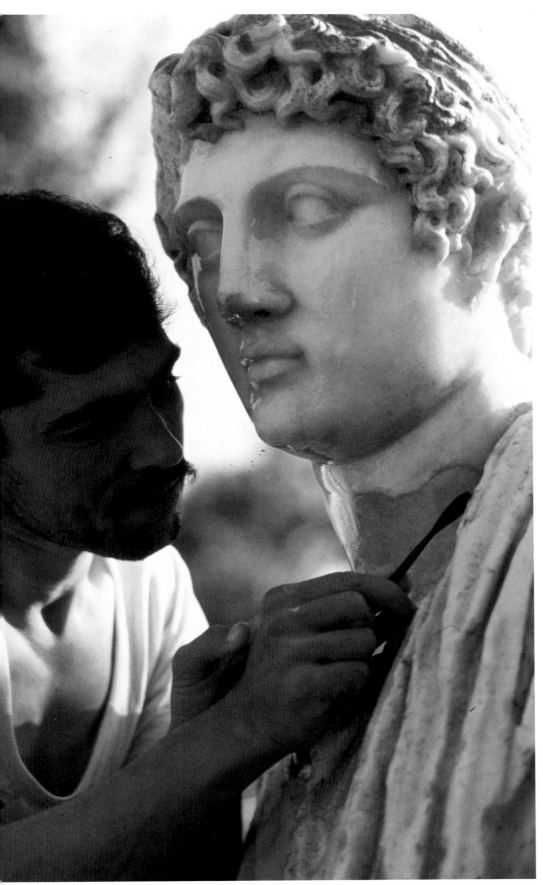

Whether in the old storage depot or in the still unfinished Museum halls, the cleaning, resetting, restoration and rejoining of countless remarkable Aphrodisian works of art went on unabated in the weeks preceding the Museum's inauguration.

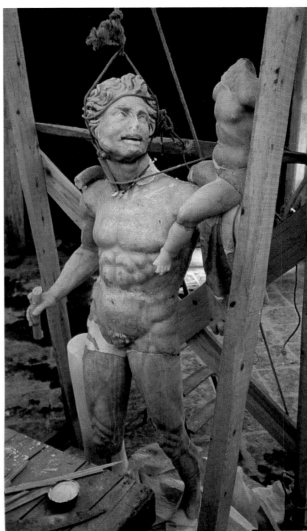

The Sebasteion

Our most interesting and fortuitous discovery was made in a house foundation, close to the surface, near the eastern edge of the Agora, not far from our excavation headquarters. Intriguing relief fragments were encountered first, and were found to correspond with other pieces haphazardly recovered in or near the village houses of the area in previous years. The outcome of a small sounding was so thought-provoking that it was decided to extend this into two larger trenches.

These excavations and concomitant study activities between 1980 and 1983, produced an extraordinary quantity of large relief sculpture and gradually brought to light the well preserved remains of a rare building complex which these reliefs had once decorated. This complex we came to identify, tentatively, as a 'Sebasteion'.

The word is derived from the Greek 'Sebastos', equivalent of the Latin 'Augustus' and means a place devoted to the cult of the deified emperor Augustus-Sebastos, and his Julio-Claudian successors. This was, by implication, a building devoted to the Imperial cult, since all Roman emperors eventually assumed the names or titles of Augustus or Caesar. Reference to a Sebasteion at Aphrodisias was known from an inscription in the *Corpus Inscriptionum Graecarum* (2839, 1.2.), but this did not provide any precise information concerning its location.

The Sebasteion was situated in the south-eastern part of the city,

The sudden revelation of the presence of the unique and extensive first-century AD monument that came to be known as the Sebasteion was an exciting sequel to the inauguration of the Museum. This lavishly decorated complex of structures provided additional proof of the originality and skill of Aphrodisian sculptors in combining architecture and sculpture. Many of the relief panels of the Sebasteion were found miraculously close to the surface of the village street *(below right)* that skirted the excavation headquarters and had covered them for many centuries. These reliefs included representations of vanquished peoples or tribes *(below)* and other allegorical figures.

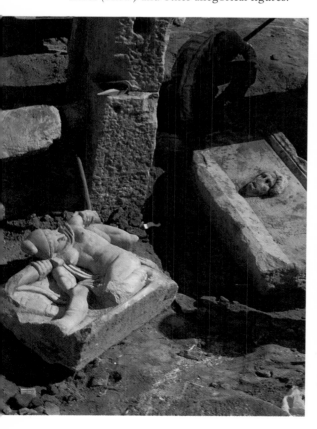

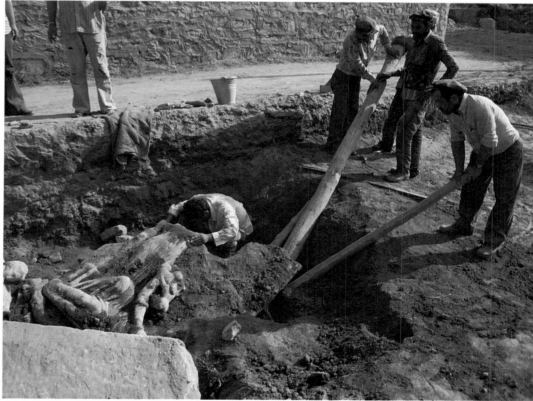

to the east of the Agora. Its plan did not show any alignment with the visible remains of the Agora, nor with any other structure so far known; its orientation is essentially east-west. This is not unusual since the available evidence has revealed many such diversities in the city plan of Aphrodisias. Its only regular sector appears to be the Agora complex itself and its two large porticoes.

In its present, still not entirely excavated state, the Sebasteion consists of two parallel porticoes about eighty metres long. These porticoes faced one another, but were separated by a paved area, about fourteen metres wide, which may have acted as a sort of processional way. At the west end of the complex, these terminated in, or were joined into, a propylon. This gateway was arranged somewhat irregularly in relation to the porticoes. It was not perpendicular, but formed an obtuse angle against them. At the opposite end, a flight of ascending steps was added, probably in early Byzantine times. These bridged the area between the porticoes — again irregularly — and led to a platform to the east. A temple or shrine was probably located here on higher ground, dominating the porticoes and the processional way, and thus the whole complex. Traces of its crepis and its stylobate as well as a number of column drums, Corinthian capitals and entablature (including fragments of an inscribed architrave) were recorded in the exploration of this area in 1982. Unfortunately, the presence of a village house has delayed further investigations here for the time being.

Of the two porticoes, the south one was discovered first, in 1979.

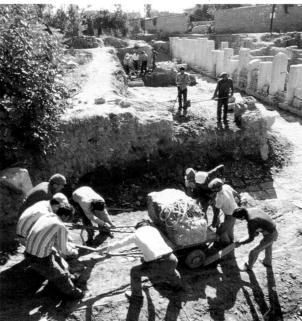

The excavation of the Sebasteion *(above)* was the chief focus of operations after 1979. The complex appeared to have been inserted in a relative elongated area east of the Agora and consisted of two parallel porticoes about fourteen metres apart *(see plan below)*.

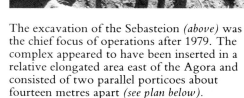

APHRODISIAS
SEBASTEION AND VICINITY

N

North portico

South portico

0   10   20 m

In many ways it is the better preserved of the two. Continued study indicated that the façade looking toward its counterpart to the north resembled a kind of stage façade and consisted of three superimposed storeys of half columns rising to a height of about ten metres.

The lowest columns, most of which were found *in situ*, were Doric; those of the next storey, all of which had fallen, were Ionic; and those of the topmost storey were Corinthian. Large decorative relief panels and other elements were inserted between the intercolumniations of the second and third storeys. The ground storey revealed a sequence of repeated units, composed of one wider central intercolumniation flanked by two narrower ones. This arrangement seemed to suggest a central doorway and two window areas on either side. The ground plan of the portico echoed this partitioning. The original purpose of these chambers is so far unclear, but it is probable that the additional screen separations were added in Byzantine times, when the Sebasteion may have been used as a market, or perhaps even as a living area. Heavy central pillars in the interior, however, undoubtedly belong to the original construction.

The parallel north portico was discovered in 1981 and gradually excavated in 1982 and 1983. Its general appearance — a three-tiered

On higher ground, perhaps a podium at the eastern end of the well-paved processional way between the two parallel porticoes, stood the temple of the Sebasteion. As the results of earthquakes in the later fourth century AD, which caused havoc to the water table and canalization of the area. The temple area may well have been threatened by flooding waters from the eastern mountains. Consequently, emergency measures in the form of a series of drainage channels and terracotta pipes were engineered in and around the structure in order to evacuate these waters in a westward direction. These were concealed beneath a platform and the series of steps descending to the processional way.

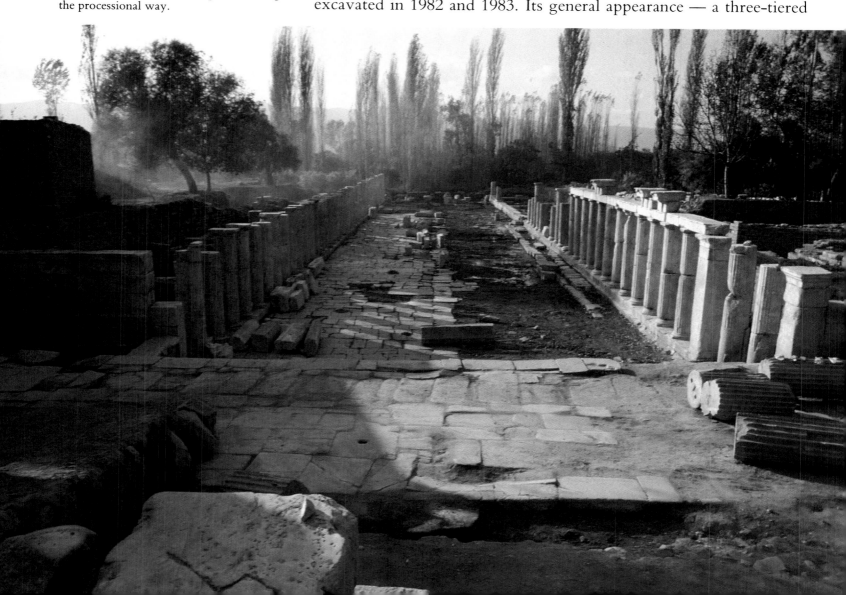

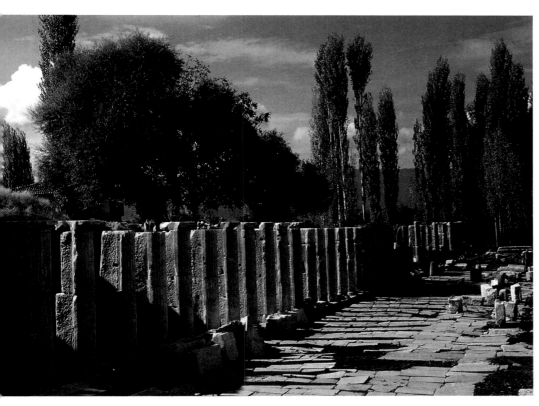

The façade of the south portico *(left)*, dedicated by one family, displayed three storeys of half-columns, which were Doric, Ionic and Corinthian in ascending order. The north portico *(below)* dedicated by another family, showed subtle but clear differences from its southern counterpart, although it echoed its essential lines.

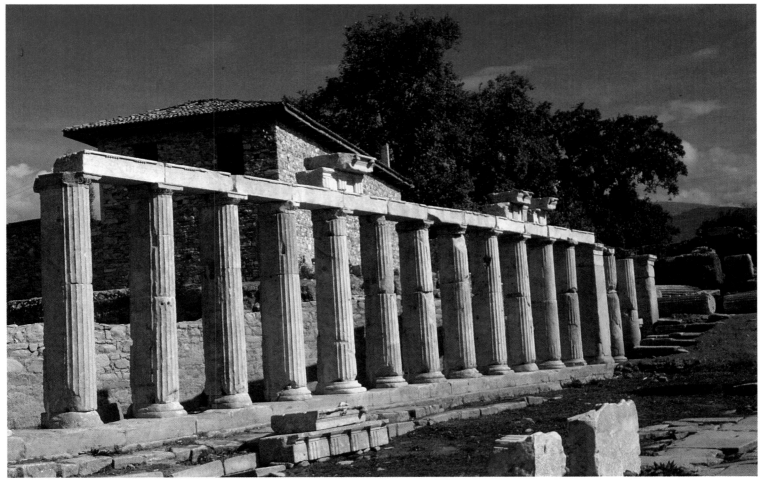

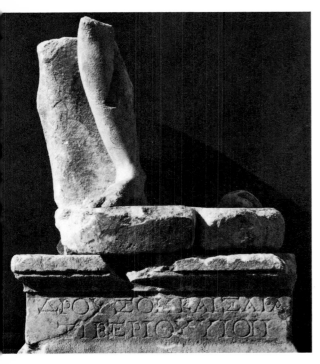

The west end of the Sebasteion was closed off from a street at lower level by an elaborate monumental gateway, of which only elements remain *(below)*. This propylon was set slightly out of alignment with the porticoes and featured two pylons each with two storeys of columnar niches connected at either side to the porticoes with intervening flights of steps.

façade (opposite that of the south portico), and the arrangement of orders — was essentially similar to the south portico. There were, however, certain marked differences. The Doric half columns of the ground storey were entirely fluted, rather than of the 'Pompeian' type which is characterized by a smooth lower drum. Its inter-columniations were equal and did not vary. Consequently, there were no unit divisions, at least none visible on the façade. The internal arrangement did have chamber units, but Byzantine modifications may have been responsible for creating them. Also, the crepis and stylobate of this portico were higher, and its eastern end, near the flight of ascending steps of later date, gave the appearance of a propylon-like façade, composed of two partly fluted Doric columns, flanked by two antae (square pillars).

Several architectural details in the west end of this north portico reveal repair work that perhaps took place after damage caused by an earthquake in the first century. On the other hand, archaeological evidence suggests that more serious problems affected the whole complex at a later date, possibly in the second half of the fourth century. The earthquake that damaged the Odeon and the Theatre also affected the Sebasteion. Here, as elsewhere in the city, flooding occurred after the water table was disturbed and some canalisations and water-channels were destroyed. To try to stem the inundations, a number of new evacuation channels were created in the processional way, and also in the platform above the steps. The flight of steps at the east end of the complex was devised at this time to conceal a number of conduits and canals and evacuate the waters that may have endangered the Temple itself. The effects of the fourth-century flooding and changes in the water table are still noticeable in the area of the propylon and have been exacerbated by the irrigation channels dug by farmers owning land in the area of the

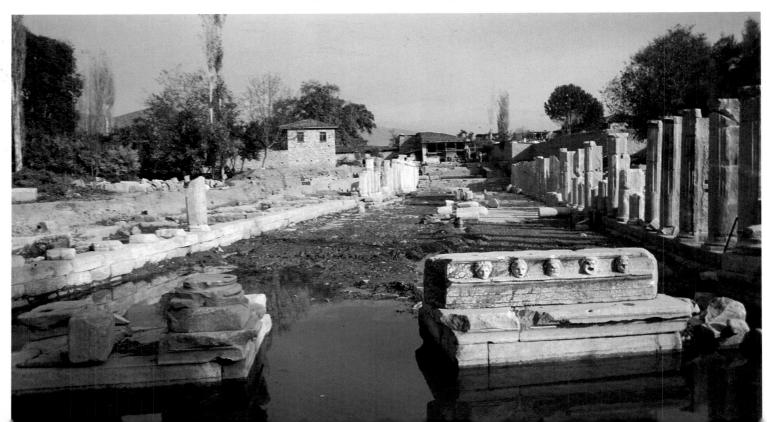

Agora. The function of the Sebasteion was probably also changed in the fourth century. It may have been used briefly as a market.

The final disaster affecting the complex was also caused by an earthquake of even greater intensity. This must have occurred in the first half of the seventh century, in the reign of Heraclius (610-641). Beside the Sebasteion, it destroyed the stage of the Theatre, the Odeon, and the so-called Agora Gate at the eastern end of the Portico of Tiberius.

Recent excavations in the area of the propylon have provided interesting data concerning this section of the Sebasteion. The gateway consisted of two units, or pylons, that were placed in the width and at the end of the processional way, and included three flights of westward descending steps in between. These acceded to a street or to the nearby Agora, but also served to join the adjacent ends of the north and south porticoes.

The façade arrangement of the propylon featured columnar aediculae in two storeys. The first order consisted of Ionic columns with reed-fluted drums, the second of regular Corinthian columns. The eastern side, facing the interior of the complex, was essentially linear and unbroken, probably for structural as well as aesthetic reasons. The western side, however, facing the Agora, offered a view of meandering aediculae, accentuated by a system of 'half' or broken pediments. At one time, statues on bases were placed in the niches. Due to flooding, the fragments and five inscribed bases of these statues were recovered only with great difficulty. They included the remains of statues of Lucius and Gaius Caesar, the two grandsons of Augustus; of Drusus Caesar, son of the emperor Tiberius; of Aeneas; and of Aphrodite herself. The goddess was described, interestingly, as the "ancestral mother of the divine Augusti" (*prometor ton theon Sebaston*).

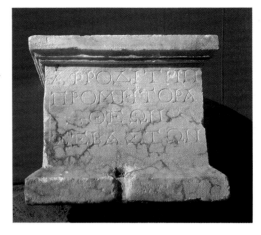

Many inscribed statue bases and fragments were recovered from in front of the gateway and undoubtedly must have been at one time fitted into the niches in the two pylons. Inscriptions included the names of a great many members of the Julio-Claudian Imperial family - for example Drusus, son of Tiberius *(opposite top)* as well as that of Aphrodite Prometor *(above)*. The frieze of the first storey of the gateway displayed superbly executed theatre masks, *(below left)* including one of a head crowned with ivy leaves, probably representing Dionysus *(below right)* which is particularly outstanding.

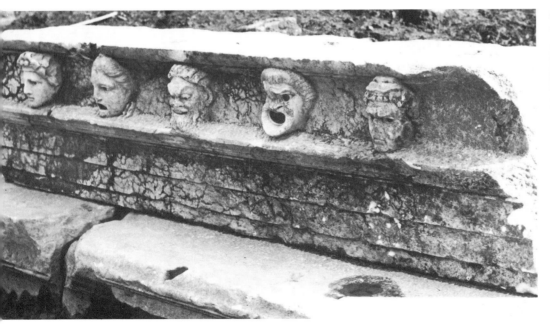

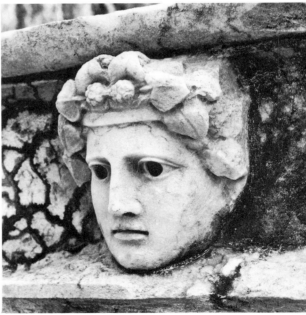

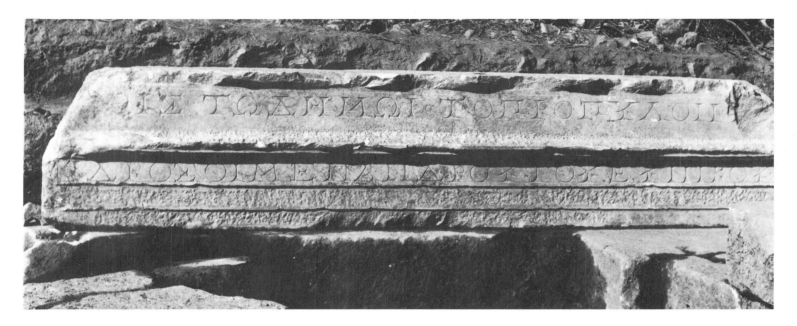

The dedicatory inscription of the propylon was cut on both the external and the internal faces of the architecture of the first storey of the building. It appears that the donors of the propylon were the same family that provided funds for the north portico.

A precise restoration of the gateway — which could prove to be one of the earliest aediculated façades in Asia Minor — is currently under way, after close analysis of most of its component parts. Particularly attractive theatre masks decorated the frieze of the first storey. The same dedicatory inscription was carved on the architrave of the east and west faces of the propylon, so that it was possible to read the identical text when either approaching or leaving the Sebasteion. The propylon was dedicated to "Aphrodite, the divine Augusti and the People", by Eusebes, Menander, their sister Apphias and her daughter Tata as well as her grandchildren. According to a further inscription discovered on the west end of the portico, the same individuals were responsible for the construction of the north portico along with the repairs to it made necessary after damage caused by an earthquake. The donors of the south portico, named in its architrave inscription, were from a different family, the most important member of which was a certain Tiberius Claudius Diogenes.

The identification and specific dates of the Sebasteion, a unique complex connected with the Imperial cult, were conveniently suggested by the remarkable combination of archaeological information — including plan, layout, stylistic considerations of its architectural and sculptural decoration — and clear epigraphic evidence. All these inscriptions point to dates in the early half of the first century AD, starting from the reign of Tiberius (14-37) and extending into those of Claudius (41-54), and Nero (54-68).

However damaged, either by human hands or their own violent collapse, the extraordinary series of panels that were inserted in the intercolumniations of the upper two storeys of both porticoes provide an unprecedented variety of unfamiliar as well as familiar mythological scenes, such as the panel showing The Three Graces (opposite). Many imperial figures were also represented in this extraordinary collection.

The most spectacular aspect of the complex was undoubtedly its lavish sculptural decoration. This consisted of large (about one metre sixty by one metre thirty), deep relief panels that were inserted into the intercolumniations of the upper storeys of the façades of both porticoes. These panels can be divided into several groups. One, particular to the south portico, was distinguished by a

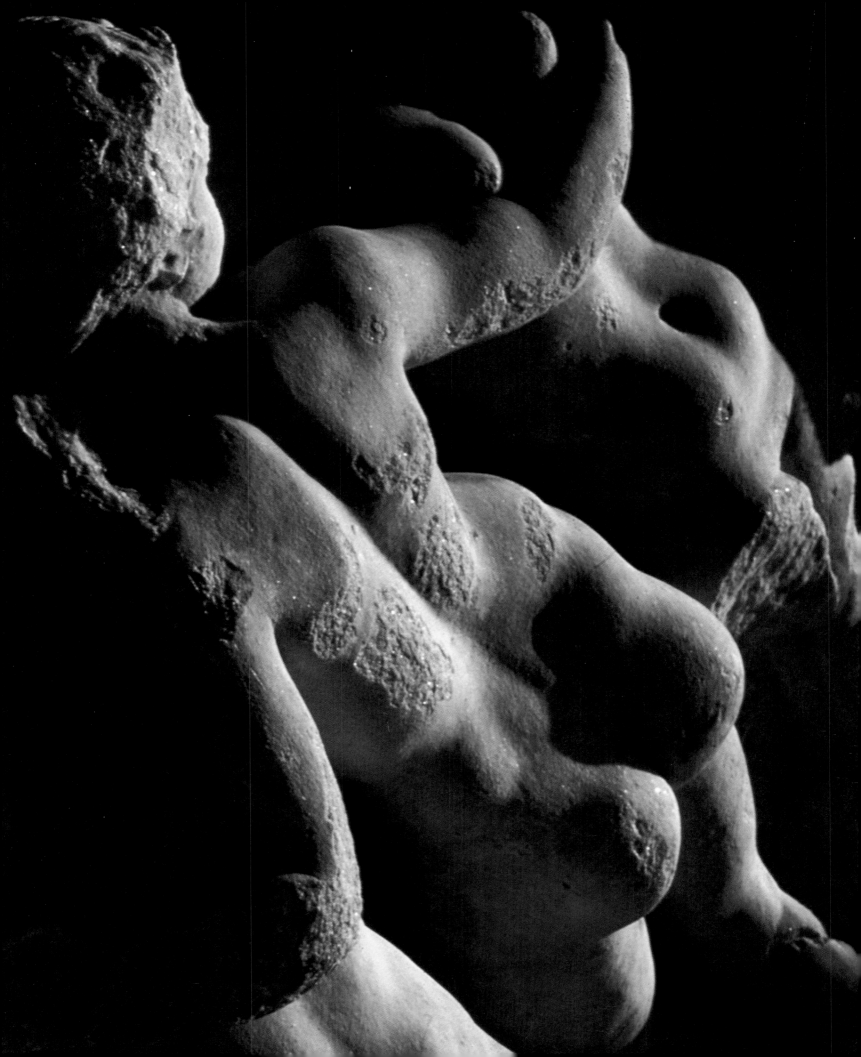

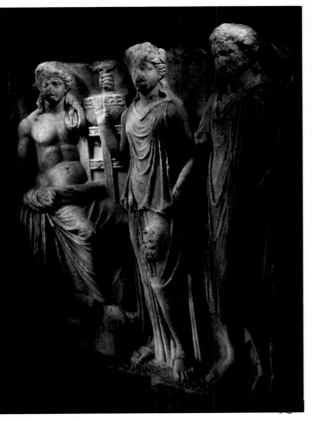

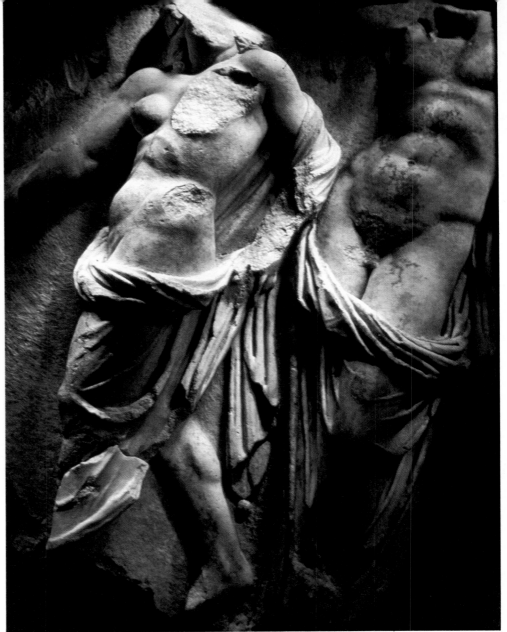

Of the sculptural decoration of the two porticoes, those of the south are better preserved. They include one series of panels characterized by a maeander-based pattern placed on the second storey of the portico. Among the scenes portrayed, one can count Apollo at his oracular shrine at Delphi attended by his priestess, the Pythia *(above)*; Dionysus preceded by walking a maenad *(above right)*; and a romantic rendition of the ill-starred Achilles and Penthesilea *(opposite far right)*.

maeander-decorated base above which were portrayed mythological scenes. These include Leda and the swan; the baby Dionysus presented to Nyssa, his nurse; Io and Argos; the Three Graces; the birth of Eros; Apollo and the Pythia at the oracle at Delphi; Bellerophon with Pegasus; Achilles and Penthesilea; and many others. As most of these panels were found fallen outside or in front of the portico, they were probably fitted on the second storey, above the window arrangements of the ground floor.

Another group, whose subject matter immediately suggested the identification of the whole complex, portrayed Augustus and other Julio-Claudian princes, emperors and princesses. The precise identities of many of the figures are still uncertain, although several can be easily recognised. The most striking is a panel showing a striding nude male figure, drapery billowing behind him as he receives the bounties of the earth and the command of the seas. This is clearly Augustus himself.

Other reliefs show princes and emperors, with trophies won from

114

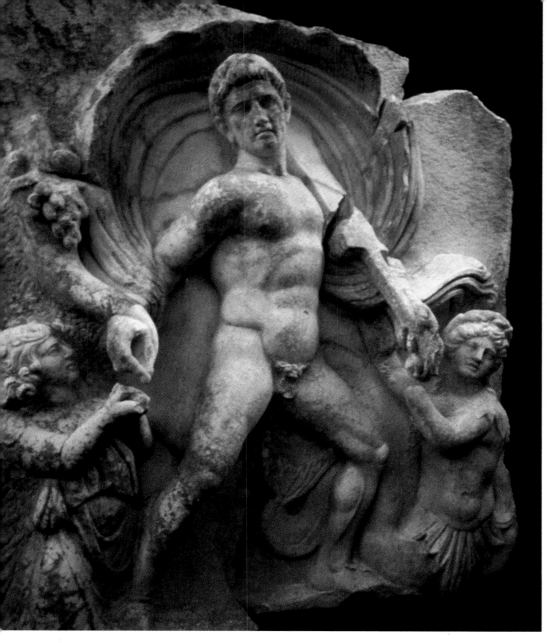

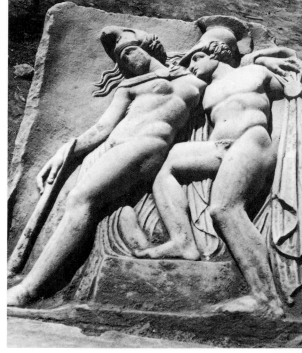

Another series of larger panels, mostly belonging to the third storey, portrayed imperial figures. The prime recipient of these divine honours was the mainstay of the Julio-Claudian dynasty, Augustus Sebastos himself, who is shown on one stunning panel *(above left)* accepting the bounties of the earth symbolized by a cornucopia with his right hand, and the command of the seas represented by an oar with his left. Other members of the family depicted include two young princes *(below left)* whose identity is not yet fully established, although they may have been Lucius and Gaius Caesar, the grandsons of Augustus.

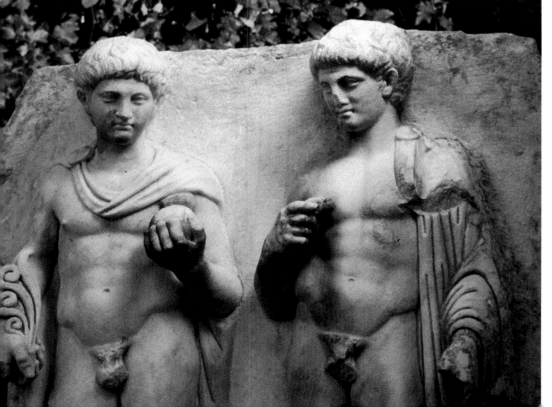

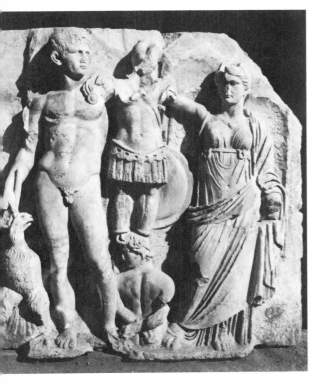

Augustus, although not identified by inscription, is again represented in a panel crowning a trophy with the help of an attractive Nike *(above)*. The imperial eagle stands at his side and beneath the trophy a bound and vanquished enemy is represented.

the enemy and the vanquished bound at their feet. Fortunately, several panels had identifying inscriptions carved on their balustrade-like bases. These identified Roma, symbolically represented, receiving the bounties of Earth (Gé), portrayed as a figure stretching out below; the emperor Claudius overwhelming a pleading personification of Britannia; and Nero overpowering Armenia. The latter panel was among several that appeared to have been battered intentionally, probably after 68 and the death of the Emperor, as part of his *damnatio memoriae*. Claudius appeared in another relief being crowned by a headless, probably symbolic, figure and shaking hands with a female figure, possibly his wife Agrippina or his deified grandmother, Livia, the wife of Augustus. Elsewhere, a relief showed Augustus crowning a trophy, with a half-figure of a bound, conquered enemy at its base, assisted by an attractive Nike to the right, and with the imperial eagle by his side.

The subject matter of the reliefs in a third group was also mythological, but did not feature a maeander-motif base. Several of these, clearly portraying pagan divinities, had been mercilessly and systematically hammered by pious Christian hands in or after the fourth century, particularly where the goddess of the city was

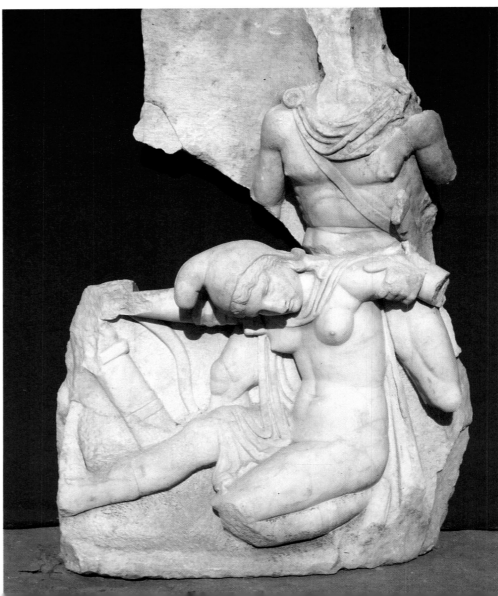

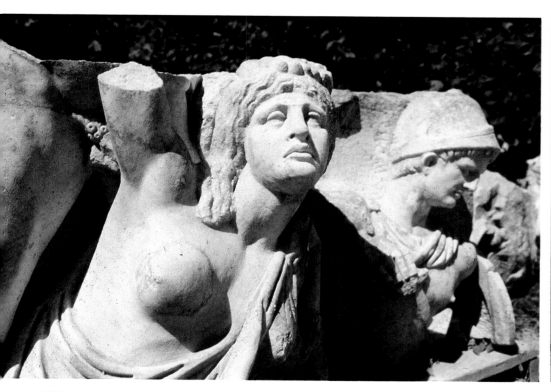

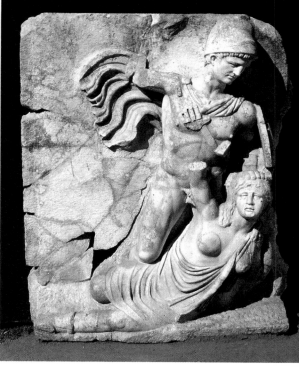

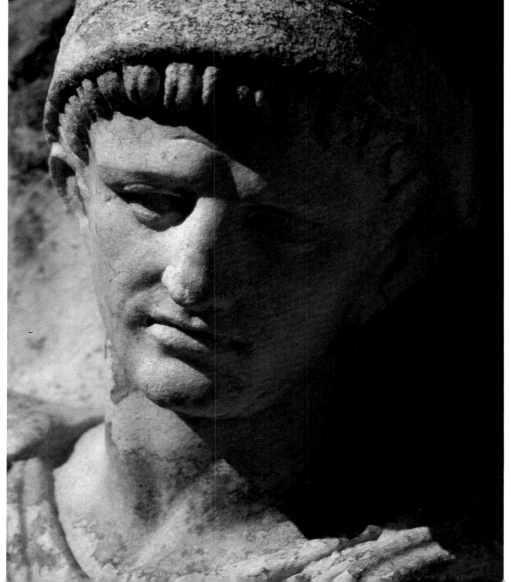

The south portico appears to have been finished or restored under the emperors Claudias and Nero. These last two ruling members of the Julio-Claudian line are clearly identified by inscriptions on the balustrades of the top intercolumniations on which they stood. Claudius and vanquished Britannia are shown in fragments *(above left)* shortly after their discovery. The characteristic melancholy expression is well portrayed *(left)*, although in the restored panel *(above)*, seen from a different angle, he appears more purposeful as he grasps the pleading Britannia by her hair, in a composition probably inspired by the late Hellenistic Achilles and Penthesilea statuary group. Not to be outdone by his predecessor, Nero is shown capturing a representation of Armenia *(opposite below)*. His head, however, has been defaced and his name erased from the balustrade inscription on which he stood.

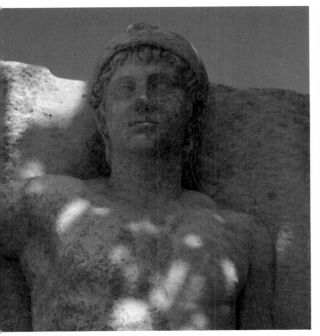

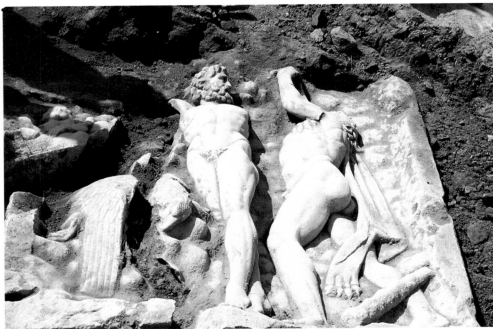

Many large panels on the south portico showing pagan deities and some mythological scenes were intentionally damaged, presumably in the fourth century AD upon the advent of Christianity. However some survived, miraculously, for reasons unknown. These include a handsome, youthful warrior *(above)*, possibly Ares, the god of war; and a portrayal of Aeneas carrying his father Anchises, and looking down at his son Ascanius with Creusa, his wife, or Aphrodite, his mother, standing sadly beside him *(right)*. The most stunning relief among these panels is undoubtedly the liberation of Prometheus by Herakles from his chains on Mount Caucasus, the tormenting bird who had constantly pecked at his liver dead at his side. This was unearthed in fragments *(above right)* and restored *(opposite)*. This original composition again demonstrates the extraordinary talents and art historical understanding of the Aphrodisian sculptors.

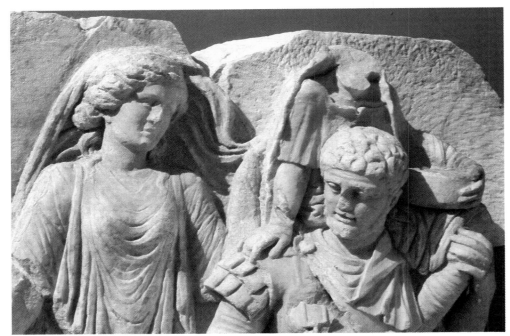

represented. Especially striking and relatively well preserved among these are the depictions of the deliverance of Prometheus from Mount Caucasus by the hero, Heracles; the flight of Aeneas from burning Troy with his father, Anchises, on his shoulder and his son, Ascanius, under the watchful protection of his mother Aphrodite; Heracles dedicating what appears to be his quiver to a herm figure of Pan; and a handsome, youthful nude warrior, perhaps Ares, the god of war.

The discovery of these imperial and mythological reliefs within the portico itself suggests that they had fallen from their original

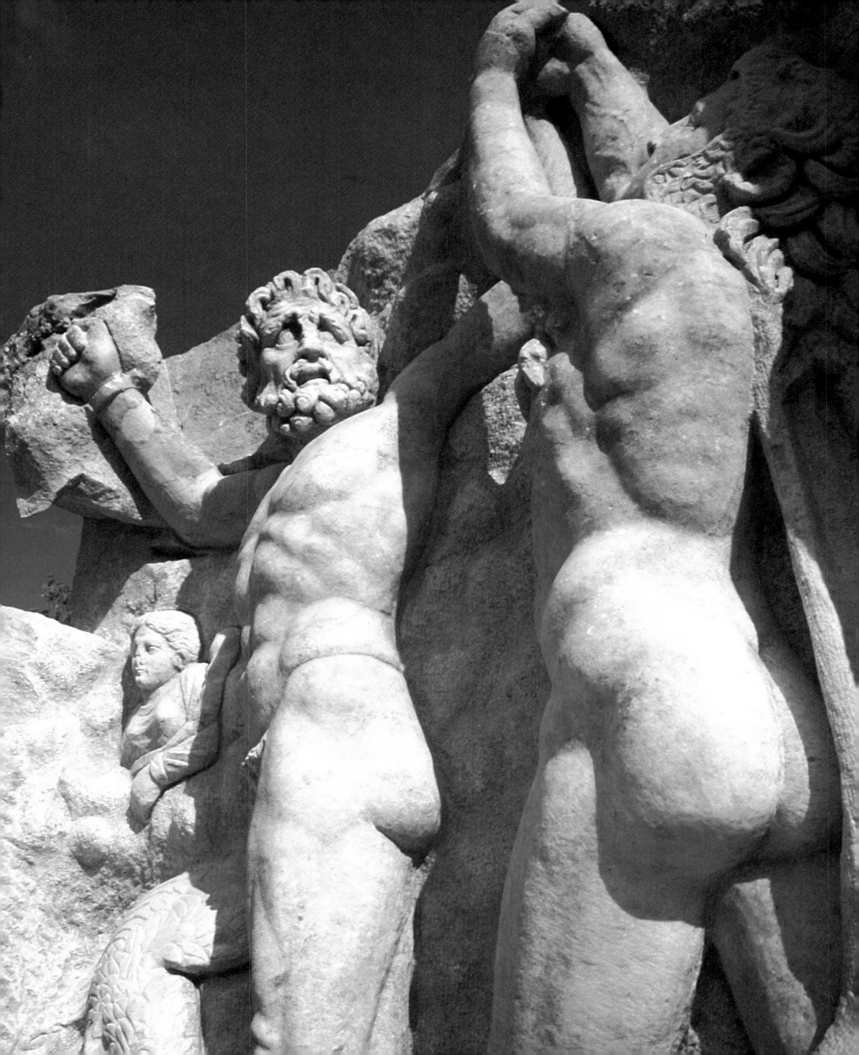

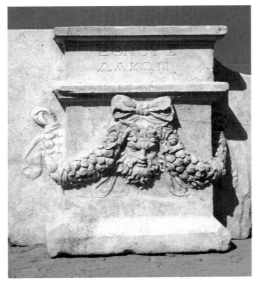

position at a considerable height and therefore must have been located in the intercolumniations of either the second storey, above the doorways, or the third. Large, coffer-type decorative elements, also recovered nearby under similar conditions, presumably acted as bases for the panels. They contained in their centre attractive relief rosettes, heads or busts of Eros, Medusa, Silenus, Helios, Selene and others.

The north portico, equally elaborately decorated with relief panels, suffered severe damage from the seventh-century earthquake. Following the collapse of this portico, many of its panels and even its architectural components, such as column drums, capitals and architraves, were taken away by the Byzantine inhabitants and used elsewhere — for instance in the fortification walls thrown up around the 'Acropolis' to transform it into a citadel, and in particular in the walls built behind the stage of the Theatre. Several of

Excavations of the north portico of the Sebasteion revealed that it had been so damaged by the seventh-century AD earthquake that some of its decorations and relief panels could easily have been removed and reused in various ways, particularly in the building of the fortification belt around the 'Acropolis'. Consequently, the full details of its relief panel decoration are uncertain. Nevertheless it would appear that the second storey intercolumniations were occupied by a group of symbolic figures representing the peoples of the empire that had been conquered by Augustus in the course of his reign. The arrangement of these figures included a *trompe l'oeil* or relief-like base consisting of an upper inscribed portion identifying the peoples depicted above and a lower moulding, with beribboned masks of various types - such as satyrs, Pan *(above)*, bearded faces *(right)*, or the like - flanked by swinging garlands. The panel bearing the symbolic figure was placed on top of this element and from below would appear like a statue standing on an inscribed base. The two bases illustrated here refer to two Balkan peoples: the Dacians *(above)* from modern Romania, and the Bessi *(right)* from Thrace.

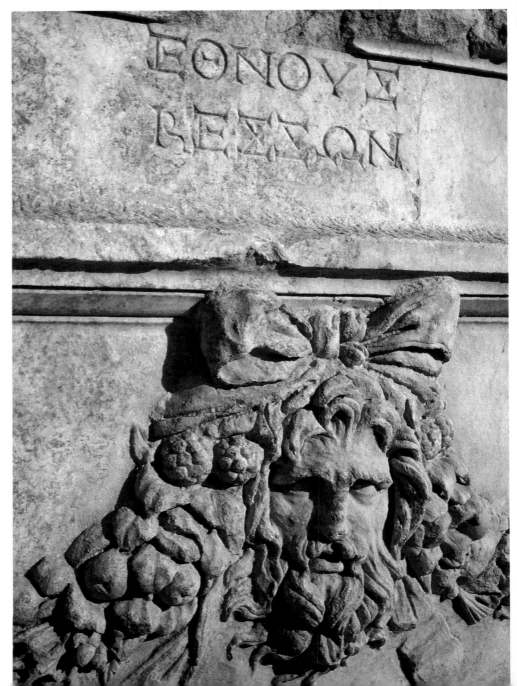

them are still visible among the blocks of the tower or 'bastion' to the north of that wall. Despite these disturbances, however, quite a few relief panels and inscribed architraves were recovered in the vicinity of the portico. Notable among the relief panels are those with 'ethnic' or 'cosmic' symbolic representations.

The 'ethnic' groups were personifications of the various peoples or tribes conquered by Augustus. Each panel consisted of two elements: one was the symbolic figure itself which stood on the second, separately carved unit, which was a *trompe l'oeil* base decorated with garlanded masks of Pan or satyrs, and with identifying inscriptions of the vanquished peoples. Among these are the names and full or fragmentary bases of at least thirteen 'peoples' including the Judaeans, the Egyptians, the Bessi, and the Dacians, as well as the people of Crete, Sicily and Cyprus, three islands recovered from Cleopatra in 31 BC, after the battle of Actium. Regrettably, more

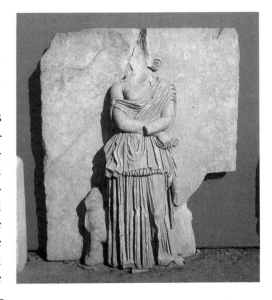

Only three complete panels with symbolic figures have been recovered. The precise identity of two of these *(above and below)* is unclear, although the militarily dressed woman *(left)* can be identified by a graffito refering to the 'Pirystae', who were located in what is now Yugoslavia.

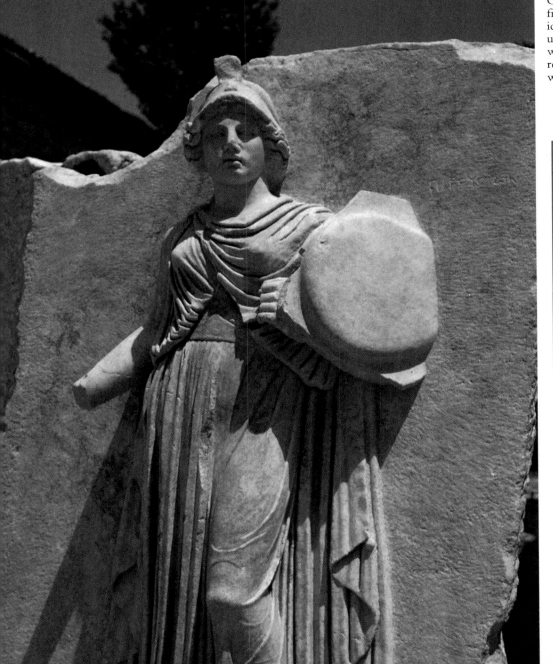

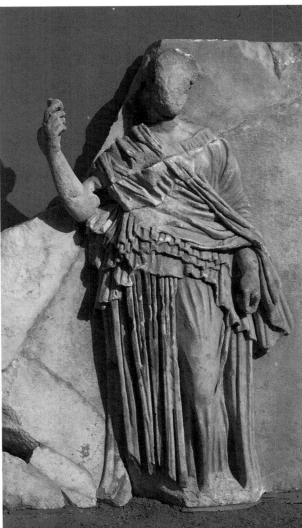

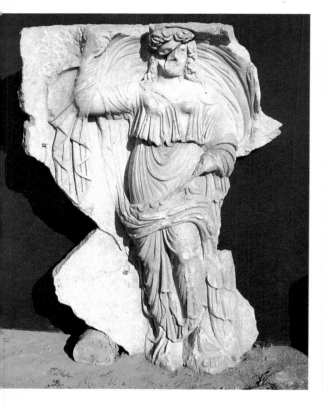

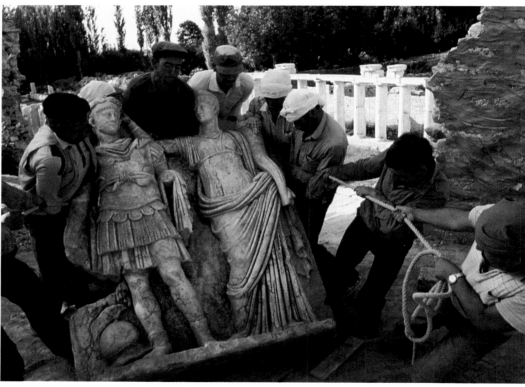

Three additional panels of the north portico of the Sebasteion are decorated with different figures. One of a pair seeming to represent 'cosmic' figures is identified by an inscription on its balustrade as *Hemera*, the Day, *(above)*. The third more elaborate panel may well have been secreted away as it was found face down within the Portico. It shows a young prince in military dress in the process of being crowned by a princess representing *Tyche*, or Destiny. The identity of these figures remains uncertain although both are obviously Julio-Claudian.

inscribed bases, or fragments of them, are extant than are the personifications that stood on top of them. Three of the latter, however, that have been found are in reasonably good condition.

Only two 'cosmic' panels have been found so far. These represent, according to their inscribed bases, the Day (*Hemera*) and the river Ocean (*Okeanos*). It is likely that these were located in the top intercolumniations.

A well-preserved relief recovered in one of the chambers of the portico shows a young prince or emperor in military dress, being crowned by a princess or empress in the guise of *Tyche* (Destiny), holding a cornucopia. Both figures are clearly members of the Julio-Claudian Imperial dynasty, but their precise identities are subject to debate, since the iconography of many of the members of that house has not yet been satisfactorily established. Candidates for the panel in question include Germanicus, Caligula or Nero for the young man; and one of the two Agrippinas for the lady.

The eastern end of the Sebasteion, where a temple honouring Augustus and his family probably stood, has not yet been fully explored. The large village house that was built over its emplacement was only recently demolished. However, several inscribed architrave blocks and other architectural fragments have been discovered close to the surface and nearby. If these have been correctly interpreted, the temple was large, in the Corinthian style, and was probably erected under Tiberius in the 20s AD.

Although the evidence is still incomplete, it can be reasonably assumed that the Aphrodisias Sebasteion exercised a significant

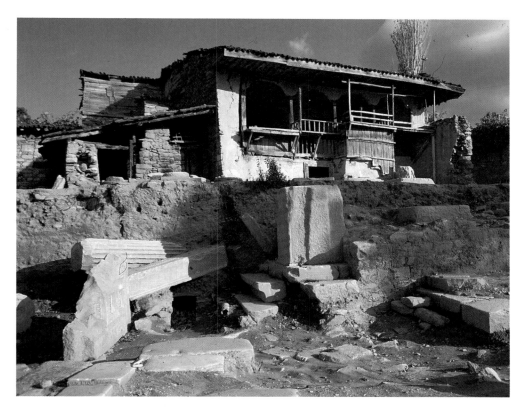

The site of the temple of the Sebasteion was occupied in recent years by a village house which was eventually dismantled. Traces found *in situ* as well as odd architectural elements found prior to dismantling indicate that this temple was finally built in Corinthian style. Inscribed architrave fragments bear the name of Livia, the wife of Augustus, and other evidence may suggest a date for its construction in the 20s AD. However, final conclusions about the character and date of this temple must wait until the full exploration of the area is complete.

influence on Roman Imperial art and architecture throughout Asia Minor and elsewhere in the eastern Mediterranean. The decorative style of the building clearly emphasized the glory of Rome, and of Augustus and the Julio-Claudian dynasty in particular. It also stressed the close mythological and historical ties binding Aphrodisias and Rome. The patron goddess of the city was, after all, the mother of Aeneas, whose descendants founded Rome and from whom Augustus and his successors claimed to have been descended. Therefore the complex would also have been intended to revere Aphrodite in connection with Augustus and his family, the *gens* Julia and other Julio-Claudians, as well as to act as propaganda for the Roman rule. In other words, the precinct may well have been an area sacred to *Venus Genetrix*, the mother goddess of the Roman people and of the Julian family. The inscribed base of the statue of Aphrodite decorating one of the niches of the propylon clearly suggests this and synthesizes such propaganda aims by referring to the goddess as the "ancestral mother of the divine Augusti."

The 'Agora Gate'

The story of the unusually close ties between Aphrodisias and Rome is still far from complete, and continues to unfold through studies and research. In 1983 for instance, continuing surveys and investigations in the so-called Agora Gate area revealed striking new evi-

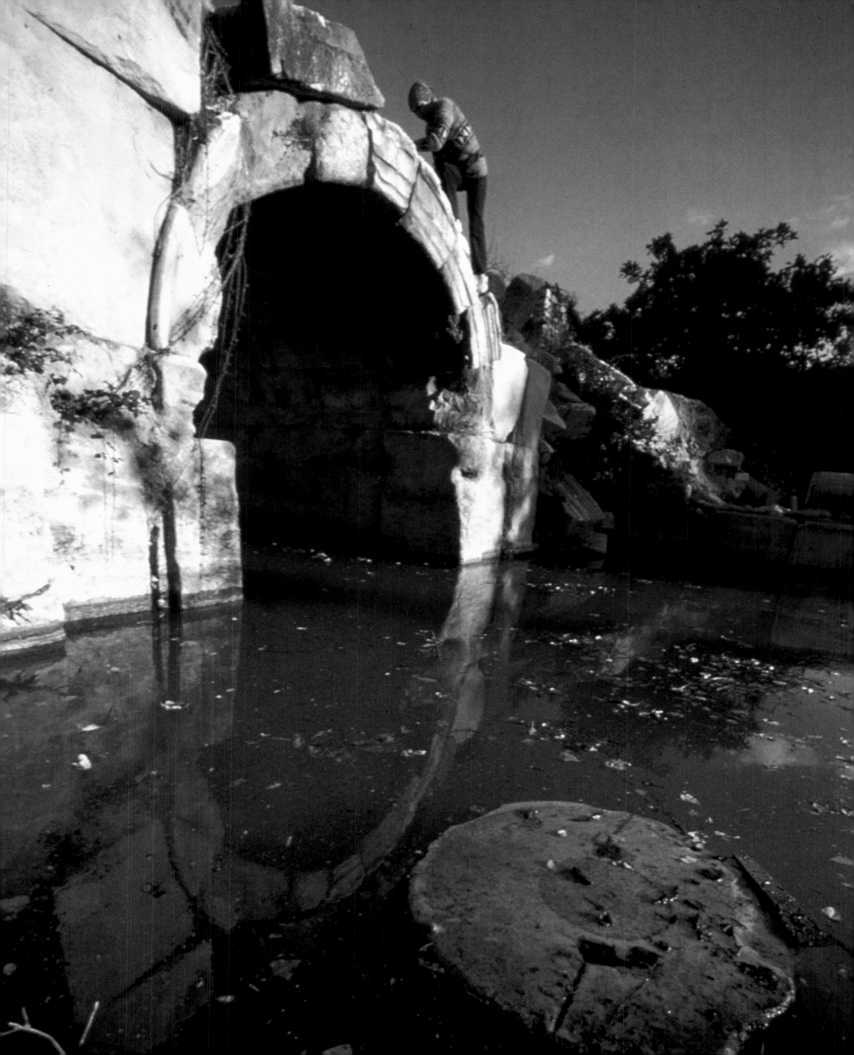

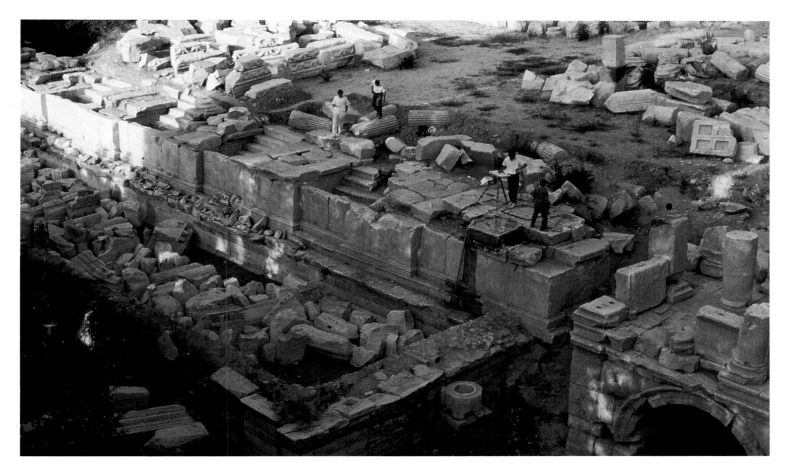

dence, although the full implications of this have not yet become clear. The impressive ruins referred to as the Agora Gate were located along the eastern width of the Portico of Tiberius (of the Agora) precisely at the opposite end from the Baths of Hadrian about two hundred metres away. The ruins were first discovered among a group of stone cottages, then sporadically and partially brought to light in 1977, 1980 and 1983. Epigraphic evidence collected during these operations indicates that the structure, which was eventually shown to consist of a huge façade, was a monumental gateway, or propylon, built in the second century. It appears to have been transformed into a fountain-house (nymphaeum) in the fifth century, following the fourth-century earthquakes which caused serious flooding in the low-lying Agora.

The façade of the Agora Gate was transformed into a fountain-house in an effort to conduct the flooding waters rushing from the east into a pool, or catch basin, through new water-pipe systems and channels built into the masonry of the building. The pool was created by throwing up retaining walls before the façade to collect the waters. Many relief panels were plundered from a neighbouring building and were set up to decorate the outward-facing wall of the pool. Among these are scenes of combat between Centaurs and Lapiths, Amazons and Greeks, and giants and gods. All of these modifications are attested to by the carving and texts of three epi-

The monumental complex constructed in the later second century AD and located at the eastern extremity of the Portico of Tiberius of the Agora appears to have been an elaborate gateway *(above)*. Inscriptions suggest that it was indeed a propylon and consisted of a massive two-storeyed columnar façade, with two projecting tower-like units at its opposite ends. Each of these featured a barrel vault *(opposite page and in the right corner of the photograph above)* topped by an upper storey of columns and leading to the east. Later inscriptions carved on the building indicate that it was transformed into a fountain house, probably in the fifth century AD, by adding a catch basin in front of its façade *(above)*.

125

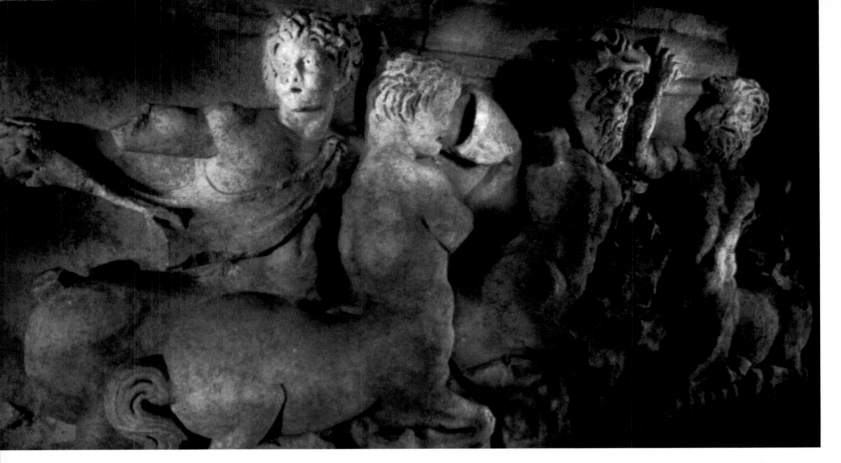

A series of relief slabs embellished with spirited scenes of feasting centaurs *(above)*, lively fights between Amazons and Greeks *(right)*, and battles between the gods and snake-legged giants *(opposite top)*, were dragged from a nearby location and utilized as odd decorative elements on top of the wall of the catch basin that was added in front of the façade.

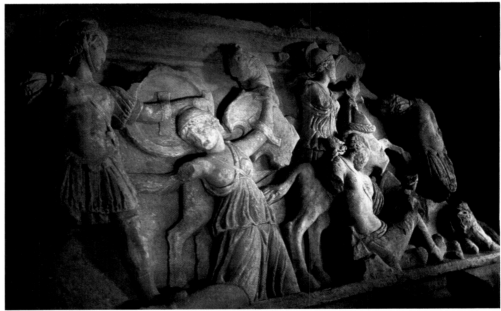

grams cut on the front wall of the façade. One of them mentions a certain Flavius Ampelius, known from other epigraphic evidence at Aphrodisias, and so probably dates from the fifth century.

Preliminary examination of the large architectural fragments and the dedicatory inscription has already provided significant information about the true identity of the agora gate. The structure was probably *not* a gateway to the Agora since it faced the Agora and did not lead to it. It is more likely that the propylon acted as an elaborate access to a still unknown complex located to the east, that is,

126

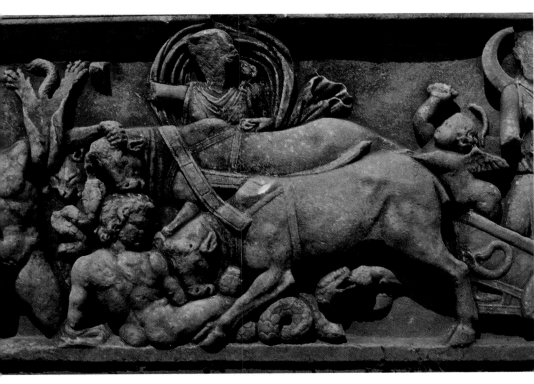

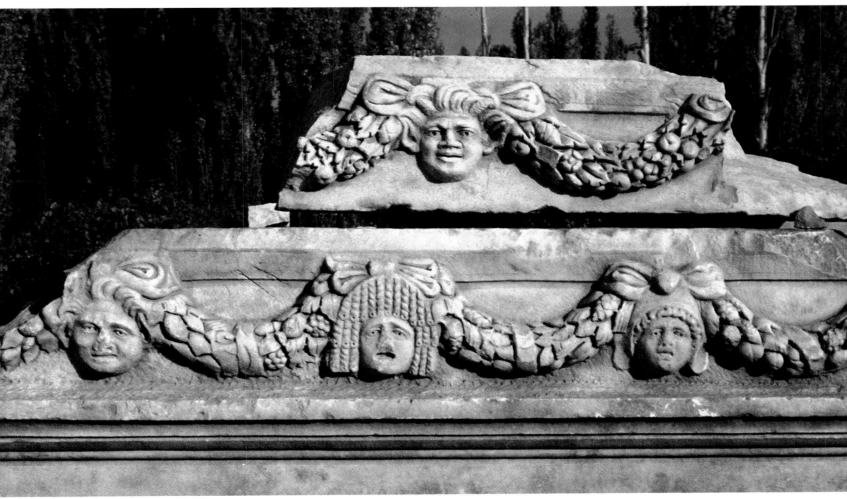

In typical Aphrodisian fashion, the frieze decoration used in the monumental complex consisted of familiar theatre masks and other faces joined by beribboned garlands.

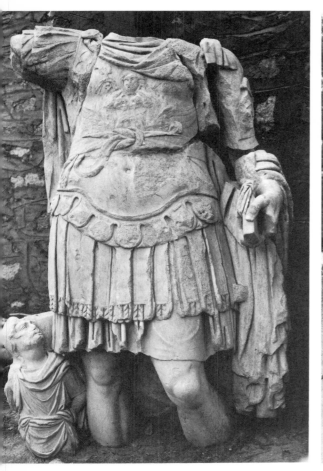

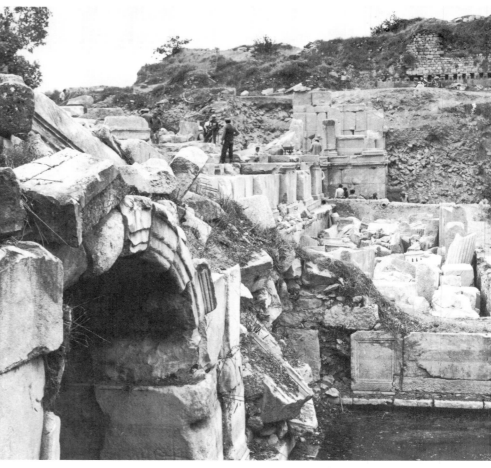

Since the main frontage of the monumental complex *(right)* faced the Agora to the west, it is unlikely that it was in fact a gateway to that public area. More probably it led to a structure or complex of some considerable significance behind - that is, to the east. It is hoped that future investigations may reveal what this may be. The statuary adorning the various niches of the façade included a colossal figure of the emperor Antoninus Pius, *(above)* identified by its inscribed base, and other figures such as the imposing statue of a handsome, toga-clad young nobleman. *(opposite page)*.

behind the façade so far investigated. The importance of this mysterious structure is implied by the monumental size of the propylon. Tentative, preliminary studies of its architectural components suggest that it was an elaborate, two-tiered arrangement with at least eight aediculae or niches, elaborate friezes of typical Aphrodisian garlands and masks, handsome statuary in the recesses, and jutting, high, tower-like units at either extremity. In short a type of towered façade.

As to the identity of the building behind the façade of the gateway, an inscription on the frieze of its first story may give us a clue. The dedication was made to "Aphrodite, the Divine Augusti and the People". This formula is known from other inscriptions at Aphrodisias, but most strongly echoes that of the propylon of the nearby Sebasteion. Furthermore, the general appearance of the Sebasteion gateway, although simpler and on a smaller scale, was not dramatically different from that of the Agora Gate. Taking into consideration several large, inscribed statue bases of the emperors Nerva and Hadrian, the recovery of a colossal statue of Antoninus Pius, with its base, and other statues of important local officials (all presumably originally located in the niches of the aediculae) it is easy to imagine that the Agora Gate may prove to be the majestic entrance to an appropriately important building or area of the mid-second century

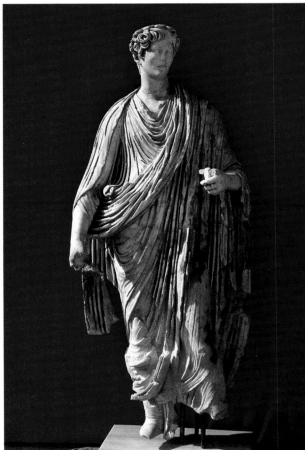

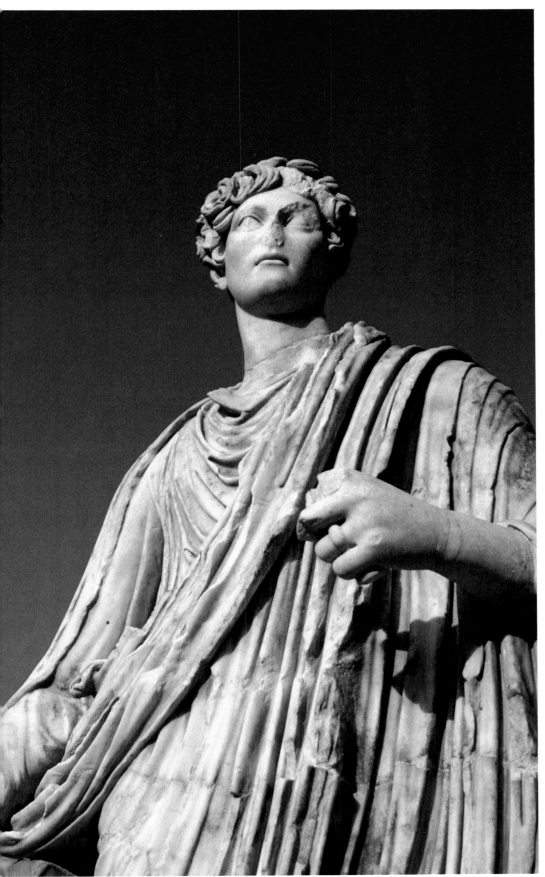

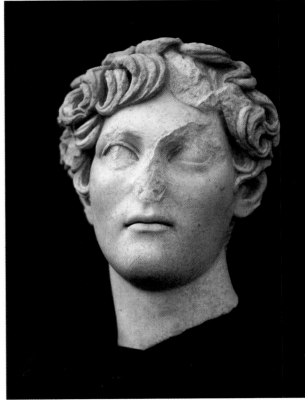

or perhaps later, also associated with the Imperial cult. Only further excavation will reveal whether or not this is the case, and until such work can be done, speculation, however tempting, is premature.

The Record of the Stones

The monuments so far described are remarkable for their often excellent state of preservation, for the high quality of their construction and decoration, and for the quantity of archaeological material that has been recovered through their excavations over the past twenty-five years. The remarkably rich array of inscriptions, coins and pottery, terracottas, jewellery, mosaic floors and fresco fragments, all of unusual interest, sheds a fascinating light on the political, social and economic conditions of Aphrodisias in the first centuries of the Christian era.

The large and significant body of inscriptions provides invaluable and detailed information not only about the history of the city, but also about the lives of its inhabitants, especially those men and women who were aristocrats or leaders of civic society and therefore intimately involved with public affairs and the government of the city. Their munificence and their service toward their fellow citizens are attested to, often over several generations, by dedicatory inscriptions on a number of public buildings.

Evidence about people of more modest status is also beginning to emerge through the study of other inscriptions. Among these are sculptors, doctors and several retired centurions of the Roman armies. Tradesmen and craftsmen also appear, from lower down the social scale. Graffiti on the seats of the Stadium, for instance, indicate that there were several craft and trade organizations that held reserved seats for the contests, shows and other exhibitions there. Goldsmiths, leather workers, and market gardeners can be identified. Furthermore, tombstone inscriptions have revealed the existence of a market overseer employed by the organization of linen workers; a head shepherd; and, at a later time, even a baker and a trouser-maker. Some epigraphic references also suggest that nails were produced at Aphrodisias from locally mined iron. Such evidence cannot, of course, give a complete picture of the economic activities of the area. It does, however, indicate that pre-industrial Aphrodisias followed a pattern that can be traced in other ancient cities.

The Synagogue

Some especially valuable information comes from a long inscription carved on an accidentally recovered pillar that must have belonged to the local synagogue. This text gives us the names and, in some cases, the occupations of some seventy Jews as well as those of over fifty other people. Some of the occupations are much abbreviated and consequently difficult to interpret with precision. Many can be identified, however, including several connected with metal working (particularly a goldsmith and bronzesmiths); with the production and processing of cloth or textiles (such as fullers and linen workers); with the food-trades (for instance, a sausage maker, a poulterer, and makers of sweetmeats), as well as several shop-keepers, a stone mason, a sheep dealer, a carpenter and what may well be a boot-maker.

The stone in question is significant for the light it sheds on the presence of a Jewish community of the Diaspora at Aphrodisias, and its relationship with the social milieu in which this community apparently thrived. It reveals a sizable group bound to its own traditions, yet one which is also remarkable for its peaceable and co-operative qualities. Its members appear to have been self-confident, accepted in the city and evidently able to attract the favourable attention of many gentile fellow Aphrodisians. Some of the latter were probably useful patrons who could help protect the interests of the Jewish community, while others seemed to have been actively involved in the affairs of the synagogue. A few were clearly proselytes.

Over fifty individuals are described as *theosebeis*, that is to say 'god-revering', and are differentiated from the rest in various ways. For instance, they did not bear biblical or Old Testament names, as the Jews did, and some were engaged in activities not consonant with Jewish law, such as city government (they include nine town councillors), athletics and even boxing. These men were probably gentiles who were sympathetic towards Judaism and who may have participated in some Jewish activities without actually becoming proselytes.

Such groups, attested to in the Acts of the Apostles and in several inscriptions from Asia Minor, have been the subject of much discussion and controversy among scholars. Thus it appears that in this context too, as in so many others, the evidence revealed by the excavations of Aphrodisias in the last twenty-five years has provided scholars with crucial information, new and important insights, and constant inspiration.

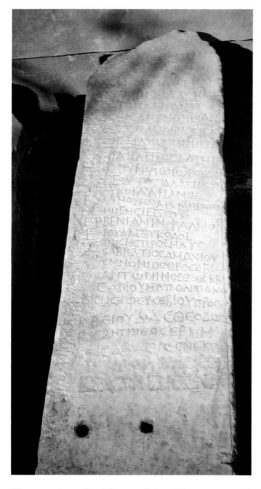

The two inscribed faces of the pillar presumed to have belonged to the hitherto undiscovered synagogue, list the names and some of the occupations of members of the Jewish community that lived in Aphrodisias and appears to have prospered there in the early centuries of the Christian era.

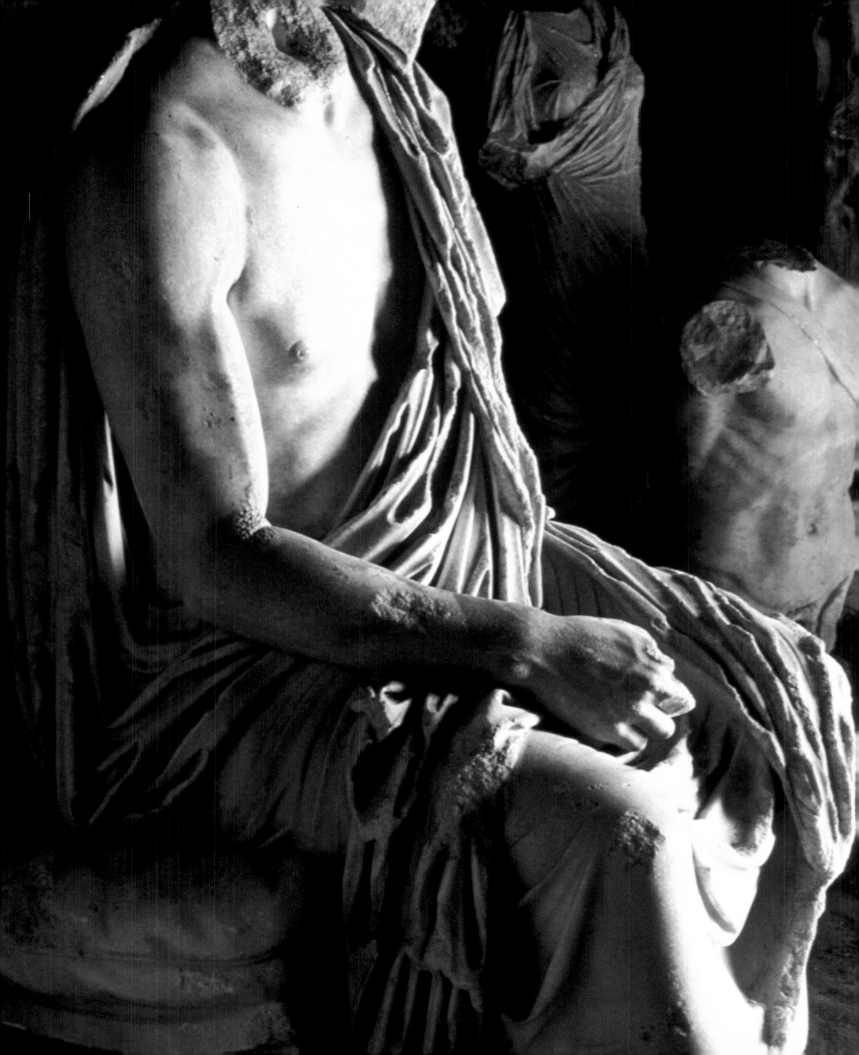

CHAPTER FIVE

Sculpture at Aphrodisias

July 21, 1979, was a memorable day for Aphrodisias. The old village square of Geyre with its hundred-year-old plane trees gradually filled with crowds who had gathered from near and far. People scuttled busily about the brand new brick and travertine-faced building that rose on one side of the square. The Aphrodisias Museum was about to be inaugurated at last. Speeches were made, welcomes and compliments were exchanged and ribbons were cut. Within minutes, visitors, villagers, guests, ambassadors and archaeologists crowded into the halls of the building to gaze and marvel at the beauty and craftsmanship of the sculpture created by the ancient Aphrodisians.

For nearly twenty years, our archaeological activities had patiently, and often against great odds, attempted to resurrect the spirit of Aphrodisias, as we unearthed magnificent statuary, handsome reliefs, unusually decorated monuments and quantities of other archaeological treasures. From the very beginning, our main priority had been the construction of a local museum to house, protect and exhibit some of this remarkable collection. It was a scholarly obligation as well as a duty to the general public. After all, it was our fascination with the marble-carving of the Aphrodisian artists that had first brought us here, and brought us back regularly every summer.

Consequently it was with justifiable pride and satisfaction that we viewed the ancient marble 'ghosts' of Aphrodisias in a suitable museum at last. These gods and goddesses, emperors and princesses, although often battered or mutilated, bore silent witness to the exceptional talents of the artists who had created them centuries ago. The high quality, sheer quantity and remarkable variety of this rich archaeological material are unprecedented. It is, therefore, now opportune to review and re-examine the contributions of the Aphrodisian sculptors to the development of Graeco-Roman art.

Unfortunately, the surviving literary texts throw little specific light on ancient art forms, and on sculpture least of all. The Aphrodisian sculptors are hardly mentioned although there is another kind of evidence about them. It consists of signed statues, fragments and bases where the name of the artist is accompanied by the ethnic adjective *Aphrodisieus*. Many of these had been found in Rome and

The exquisite craftsmanship and skill displayed by the Aphrodisian sculptors is strikingly demonstrated in this beautiful figure of a seated poet or philosopher unearthed in the Odeon.

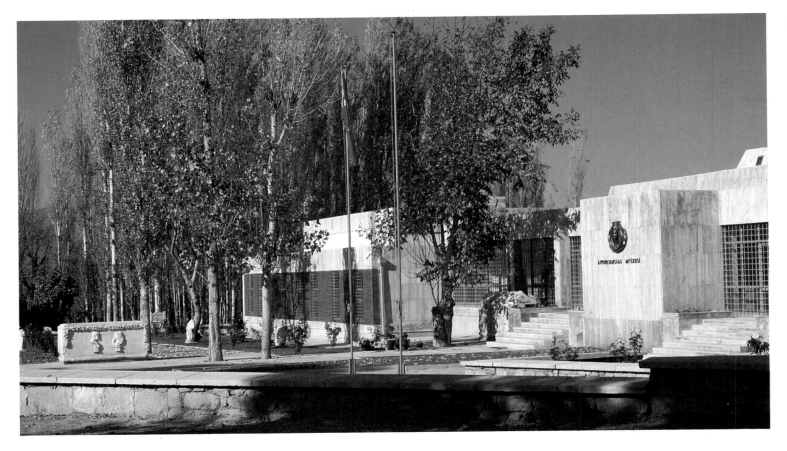

The Aphrodisias Museum, inaugurated in 1979, is undoubtedly the high point of many years of hard, painstaking work. Its exhibits of Aphrodisian sculpture extol the achievements of the Carian artists and make it one of the finest collections of Graeco-Roman sculpture in the Mediterranean.

elsewhere in Italy as well as in the Aegean, in Greece, and around the Mediterranean. The most famous were the striking figures of the old and young centaurs, discovered in the emperor Hadrian's villa at Tivoli. These bear the signatures of the Aphrodisians Aristeas and Papias. Both are now in the Capitoline Museum in Rome. Another well-known work, also found near Rome, at Lanuvium, was a handsome relief showing Hadrian's favourite, Antinous, in the guise of a divinity of the woods. In addition, there were the large number of pieces of statuary, reliefs and architectural decoration unearthed at Aphrodisias itself during the short-lived campaigns of Gaudin and Jacopi.

The Aphrodisian School

The notion that a school of sculpture had flourished at Aphrodisias was first advanced by an Italian scholar, Professor Maria F. Squarciapino, who critically examined all the archaeological and epigrahic evidence available at that time. Her study, *La Scuola di Afrodisia* (Rome 1943), was the first to champion the originality of the Carian sculptors. Unlike previous scholars, who considered them merely capable copyists of earlier masterpieces, she took the view that they were true artists who had created their own style.

134

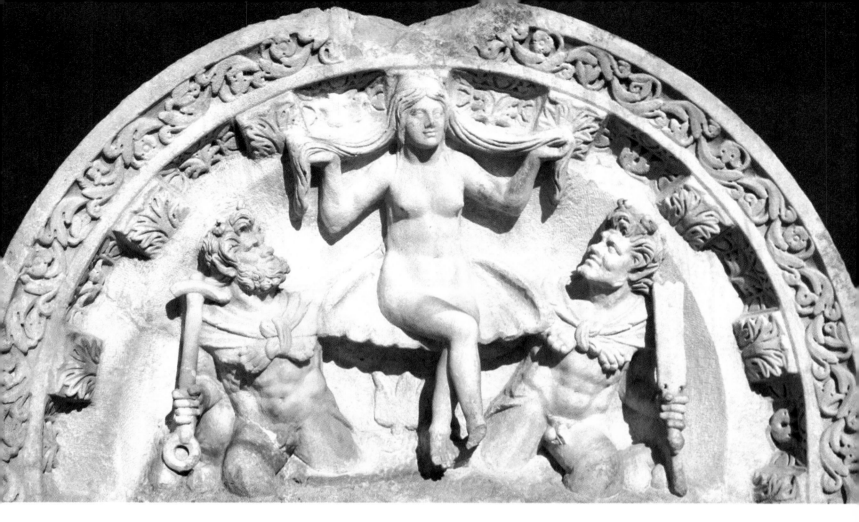

Squarciapino's conclusions have been strongly reinforced by the abundant sculptural material recovered in Aphrodisias during the present excavations. To the twenty odd names, or signatures, of Aphrodisian sculptors available before our excavations, many new ones can now be added. Notable among these are Apollonius Aster; Alexander, son of Zenon; and Menodotos. There is also fresh evidence concerning artists who were already known, such as Polyneikes, or Flavius Andronikos; and recent discoveries at Aphrodisias provide an interesting additional dimension to their activities.

The precise origins, or roots, of sculpture at Aphrodisias are difficult to accurately trace. Above all, we must consider the unusual proximity of the marble quarries, which are barely two kilometres away from the city. These played a crucial role in the development of marble-carving in the area. In comparison to other marble quarrying sites, the proximity of these to an important city was indeed remarkable and must have had great influence on the development and technical idiosyncracies of the Aphrodisians.

It is tempting to believe that some of the small 'idols' found during our recent investigations into the site's prehistory are the earliest specimens of marble-carving at Aphrodisias. However, only absolute marble-differentiating tests can prove or disprove such a hypothesis. More specific recent archaeological evidence indicates that the local marble was certainly in use during the archaic period (that is, about the seventh and sixth centuries BC). At least three

A typical relief fragment from a semicircular pediment recently uncovered in a basilica-type building to the north of the Sebasteion wittily celebrates the birth of Aphrodite. The goddess, with her legs crossed, is perched on a half shell and dries out her long wet hair in her outstretched hands. Two supporting tritons, one holding an anchor, the other an oar, gaze admiringly up at her. Both the confident treatment of the subject and the extreme care in handling decorative elements characterize the Aphrodisian 'school' in the third century AD.

fragmentary figures of crouching lions can now join the lion spout found by Gaudin near the Temple of Aphrodite as illustrations of the early use of the stone at Aphrodisias.

Surveys in the quarrying areas have revealed occasional non-Roman (or pre-Roman) methods of extracting the marble. It was in the late Hellenistic period, however, as the site developed as a city and a favoured ally of Rome, that marble-carving activities appeared to proliferate. The patronage of the Carian goddess by Sulla in about 82 BC, can be interpreted not only as a sign of increasing fame for Aphrodite, but also as evidence for other activities associated with the cult. Indeed, the construction of the Temple of Aphrodite in its final form may well have been started in the early half of the first century BC although work slowed down during the troubled years of the Mithradatic War, and again in the period of civil war which followed the death of Caesar in 44 BC. Intense work was undoubtedly resumed in the 30s BC under the influence of Octavian and his freedman Zoilos, and the Temple was completed in the last years of the century.

A prerequisite for such increased construction activities was, of course, the presence of experienced stone carvers and sculptors. Although it is plausible to assume that local craftsmen existed, such ambitious projects demanded more skilled and sophisticated artists and architects.

One theory, historically possible though difficult to prove, is that such men could have come to Caria from Pergamon. Indeed, by the end of the second century BC many sculptors and artists who had worked for the kings of Pergamon were left unemployed after the death of Attalus III, who bequeathed his kingdom and treasures to the Romans. Obviously, the Roman heirs were disinclined to pursue the artistic programmes sponsored by the Attalids; and many of the artists who had worked under the former royal patronage had to look for work elsewhere.

Some of these sculptors could easily have been attracted to Aphrodisias by commissions or, even more likely, by the excellent marble available so close to the city. They would undoubtedly have settled there eventually, in an atmosphere congenial to the pursuit of their art. Having established workshops and ateliers, their reputation, associated with that of the city as a centre of craftsmanship, would have spread, first to other parts of western Asia Minor and subsequently, beyond Anatolia to Rome, where increasing numbers of craftsmen were in demand during the later first century BC.

Ultimately their renown spread widely through the countries of the Mediterranean. The privileged status of Aphrodisias and the close ties that it had established with Rome under Octavian-Augustus and his successors could only enhance the reputation of the Carian sculptors and so help it to flourish and develop in subsequent centuries, until the decline of civic life, and of the plastic arts, in the sixth century.

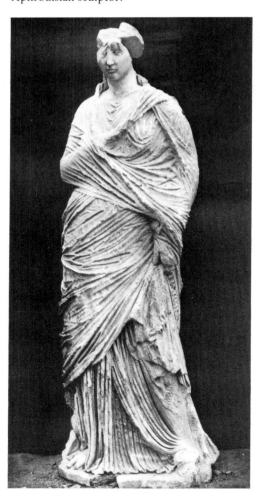

A masterfully executed draped female statue of an unknown noblewoman recovered from the Agora Gate is signed on its base by Menodotos. The quality of the workmanship in the drapery, with excellent distinction of fabric, and the sensitive rendering of the face illustrate the remarkable ability of this Aphrodisian sculptor.

Thus, the Aphrodisian 'school' thrived for a remarkably long time, and the work that came from it continued to be of a high quality. Furthermore its members succeeded in developing their style and technique over the centuries. This can be illustrated by two striking examples: one from the beginning, and the other from the end of the active period of the 'school'. The earlier work is the so-called Zoilos frieze. The later, the portrait of Flavius Palmatus.

The series of beautiful relief panels known as the Zoilos frieze were recovered partly by accident, and partly through excavation in the north-eastern sector of the city, not far from the fortification walls. Although the monument that the frieze panels decorated has not yet been located, their subject matter suggests that it must have been a commemorative one, perhaps of funerary character. The reliefs honour Zoilos, the freedman of Octavian, who was responsible for consolidating the ties between Aphrodisias and Rome and obtaining special privileges for his home town in the second half of the first century BC.

The quality of their carving and of their composition is truly magnificent. They show Zoilos surrounded by allegorical figures, each identified by an inscription. In one grouping, *Demos* (the People) greets Zoilos, who is being crowned by *Polis*, a personifi-

The most important, beautiful and also earliest masterwork of the Aphrodisian school is beyond doubt the magnificent group of relief panels called the Zoilos frieze. These reliefs, which pertain to an as yet undiscovered monument to the first-century BC benefactor of the city, show allegorical figures glorifying Zoilos. In the two panels below, the figure of *Timé*, or Honour is in the process of crowning Zoilos. *Andreia*, or Valour, attends the ceremony, holding up a shield.

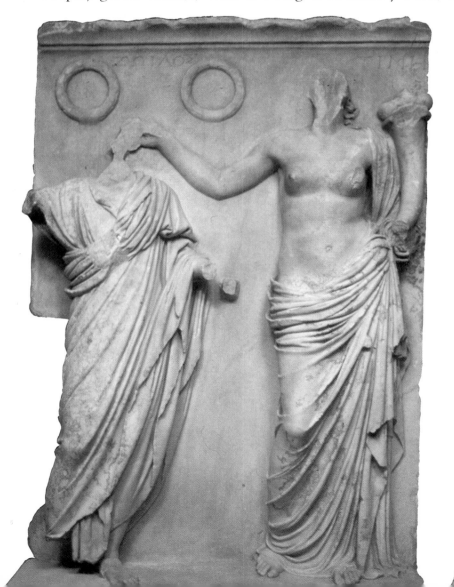
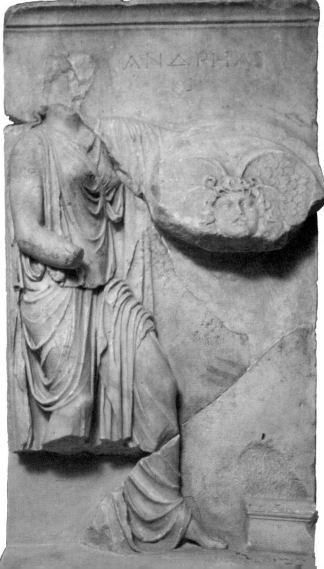

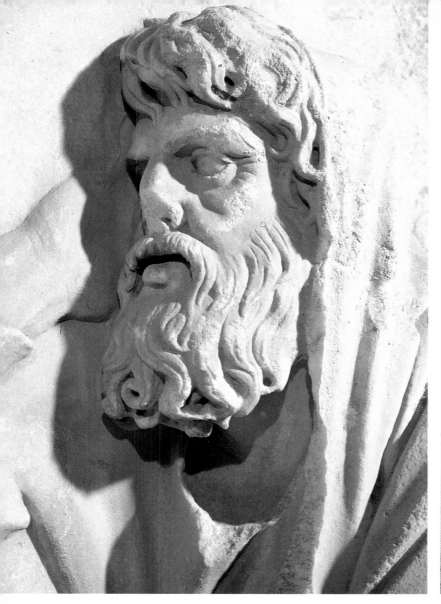

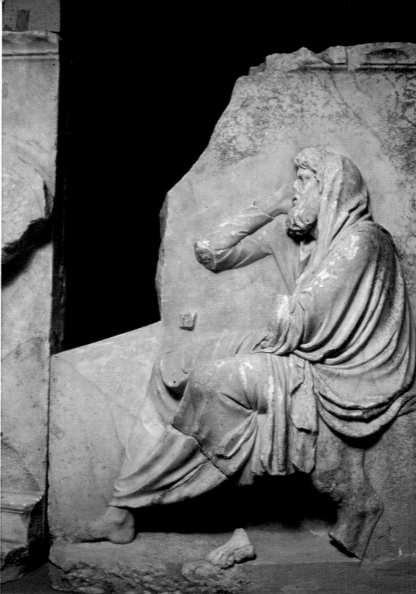

The most poignant figure of the Zoilos freize is the seated old man identified by his inscription as *Aion*, or eternity. A detail showing his face and the full figure are illustrated *(above)*. The more battered but still dignified seated figure of Roma *(opposite left)*, leaning on a shield, also comes from the Zoilos frieze.

cation of the city. The presence of hanging wreaths and a herm next to the figure of *Demos* suggest that the scene took place in or near a gymnasium. Another panel portrays Zoilos, again being crowned, this time by *Timé* (Honour). *Andreia* (Valour), *Aion* (Eternity), *Roma* and *Mneme* (Remembrance) are also represented on individual panels as a rich panoply of symbolic figures glorifying the Aphrodisian. Although some of them are more battered than others, each can be seen to have been skilfully composed and executed. The refinement of their details and their consummate elegance belie any assertion that the Aphrodisians lacked talent and originality even at the beginning of their activities.

At the other end of the period in which it flourished, the achievement of the school is no less impressive, although the style is quite different in spirit from the Zoilos frieze. The work in question has been discussed in the context of its discovery in the Tetrastoon. It is the full length portrait of Flavius Palmatus, the 'vicar' of Asiana. Created in the late fifth century, when the plastic arts were generally in a state of rapid decline, it is nevertheless an arresting work of art which reveals the continuing skill of the Aphrodisian artists.

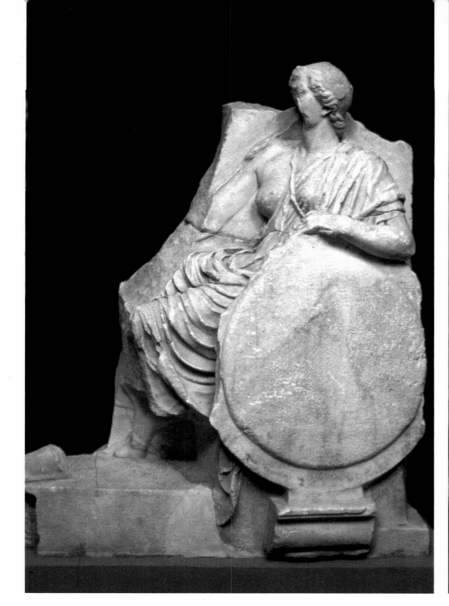

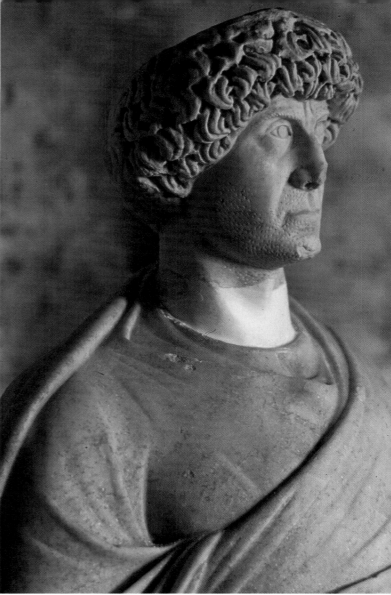

The numerous and varied sculptures found in the last twenty-five years were created in the five centuries that separate these two masterpieces. Each item confirms the impression of a school notable for its vitality and versatility. This unprecedented body of material was further enhanced by the discovery of a workshop area where many trial and unfinished items, rejects, and tools were recovered. Finally, examination of the technical idiosyncracies and quarrying habits of the Aphrodisians add another fascinating dimension to our understanding of their achievements, as well as to our appreciation of the history of ancient sculpture in general.

At the opposite end of the time span in which the Aphrodisian 'school' flourished, the late fifth-century portrait statue of Flavius Palmatus stands supreme. Although totally different in style and spirit, this masterpiece of portraiture still shows the extraordinary craftsmanship and ability of the Carian sculptors.

Conclusions

By combining all of this new evidence with conclusions already reached by Professor Squarciapino, it is possible to draw up a profile of the Carian sculptors and to summarize their main characteristics and contributions to Graeco-Roman art.

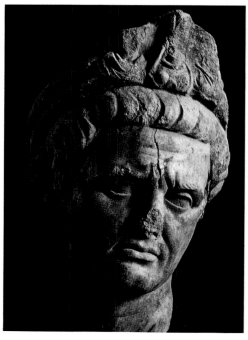

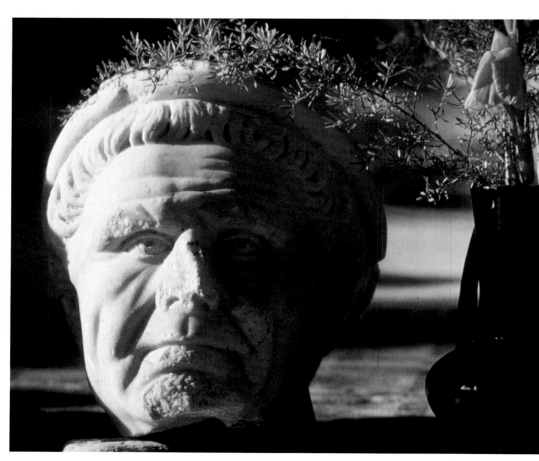

The mastery of the Aphrodisians in portrait sculpture is exemplified in many pieces such as the Flavian priest *(above)*, the Trajanic bust *(below)* and the stunning fourth- and fifth-century AD likenesses *(above and below right)*.

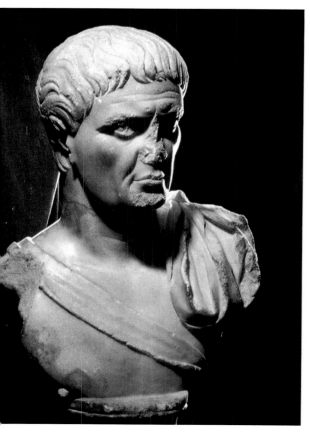

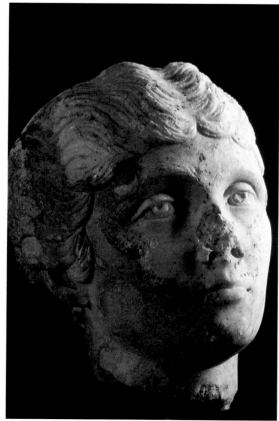

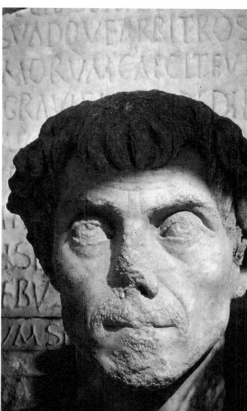

I. Their most striking achievement clearly lay in the field of portraiture. Whether Julio-Claudian, Flavian, Antonine, Severan or Constantinian, their creations stand out even among acknowledged masterpieces of ancient portrait sculpture. Especially arresting are the penetrating character studies of the later empire (fourth and fifth centuries), such as the portraits of Flavius Palmatus and the *chlamydati*, those high officials so elegantly wrapped in their long cloaks (*chlamys*), or of their female counterparts.

II. Although perhaps not originally conceived by the sculptors of Aphrodisias, much architectural decorative sculpture was carried to such high levels of imagination, sophistication and perfection that certain motifs and types became closely identified with them. The intricately executed 'peopled scrolls' pilasters of the Hadrianic and Theatre Baths and the ubiquitous mask-and-garlands friezes, were handled with consummate skill. The masks and other similar heads that adorn the frieze represent a remarkable repertory, and are often skilful variations on the models of known sculptural types which nevertheless retain a typically Aphrodisian flavour.

III. Like their Hellenistic predecessors, especially those at Pergamon, the Aphrodisian artists reflected earlier styles, themes and traditions associated with classical sculpture. Despite this eclecticism, they almost always maintained a spirit, originality of approach

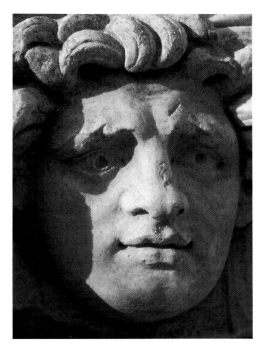

Although by no means an Aphrodisian invention, the-mask-and garland frieze used so frequently, effectively and inventively by the Aphrodisian school became closely identified with it. These two examples illustrate the genre.

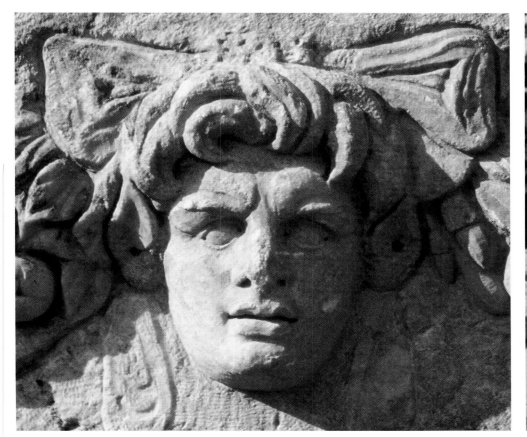

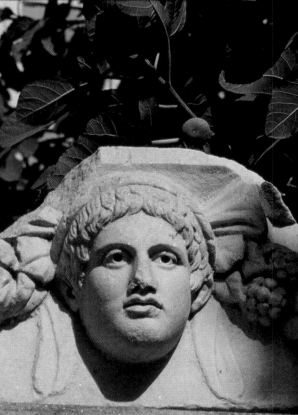

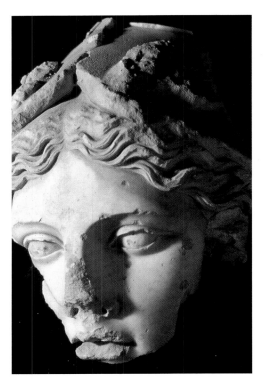

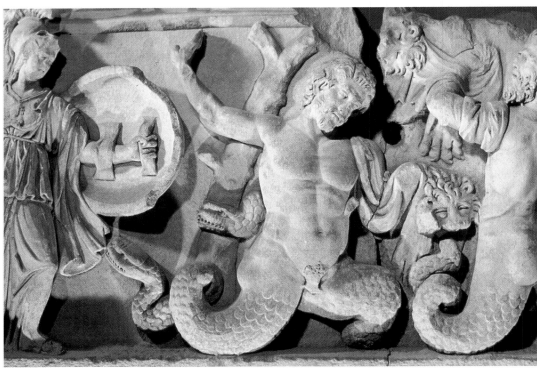

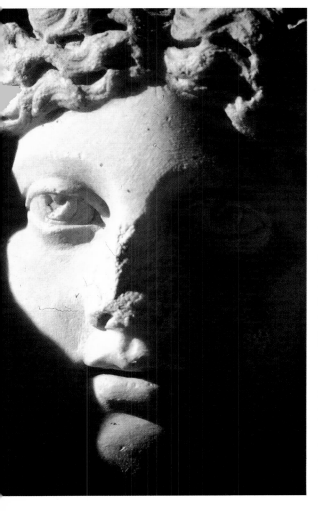

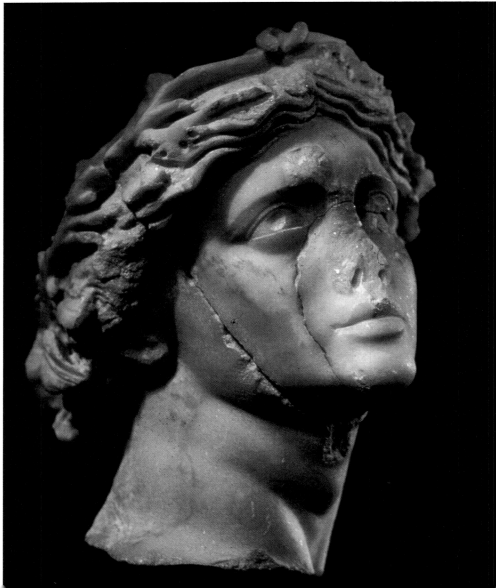

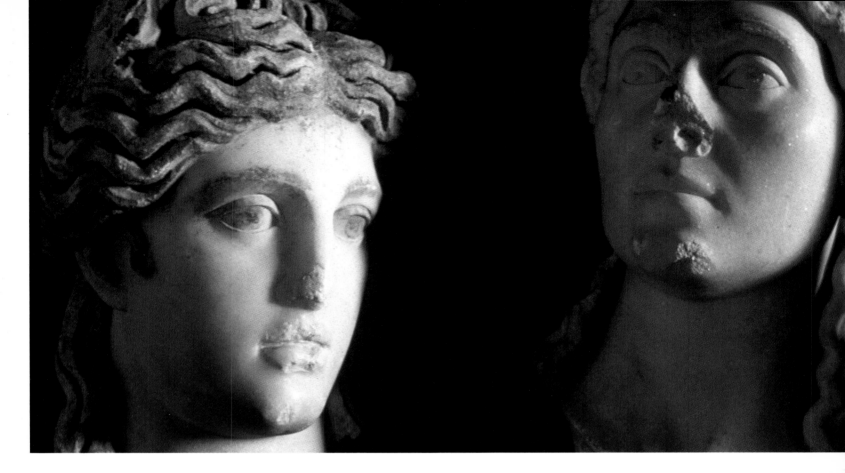

and stylistic blend that was all their own. The reliefs portraying battles between gods and giants (Gigantomachy), Centaurs and Lapiths (Centauromachy) or Amazons and Greeks (Amazonomachy) and other subjects, that have been found in the Agora Gate excavations, bear eloquent witness to a sophisticated appreciation of the great sculptors of the past. This is also true of the masks and heads that were used in architectural friezes. Groupings and composition in some of these may recall classical Attic traditions, yet other details emphasizing pathetic expressions and elaborate 'baroque' themes are reminiscent of Pergamene art. The numerous panels that decorated the Sebasteion (for instance the liberation of Prometheus by Heracles; Leda and the swan; and several Nike figures) display similar 'baroque' trends. They also echo fifth-century classical traditions and idiosyncrasies such as the portrayal of a youthful warrior, or Ares; and the representation of Demeter and Triptolemus. Another neo-classical work is the beautifully executed figure of a young athlete found in the Theatre stage and inspired by a statue by Polykleitos, the fifth-century BC Peloponnesian master.

IV. Small sculpture for domestic and ornamental purposes was created in abundance. Some may have been intended for the export market; such pieces often reflect the overblown, so-called 'rococo' style of Hellenistic sculpture. Examples include the seated Aphrodite, legs crossed, as she dries her hair — a motif repeated in a beguiling birth of Aphrodite, executed in deep relief as a semi-circular pedimental decoration. Another is a sculpture of Pan extracting a thorn from the foot of a satyr (the 'spinario'). There are also

The Hellenistic affinities of the Aphrodisian 'school', with Pergamene, barogue and neo-classical characteristics, are vividly illustrated in the skilful use of Gigantomachy friezes *(opposite above right)*; a pathetic head, possibly of Apollo *(opposite below right)*; and two traditional representations of divinities, such as the Athena *(opposite above left)* and Apollo *(opposite below left)*. The exquisite head of a classical Apollo *(above left)* and the strong portrait of a second-century AD lady *(above right)* formed an extraordinarily contrasting pair in the penumbra of the old storage depot shortly after their discovery. They further demonstrate the extreme versatility of the Carian sculptors.

Seen out of context the cheekily crossed legs of the Aphrodite figure *(opposite)* underline the 'cheesecake' character of the pose of a similar figure of the goddess in a third-century small semicircular pediment *(below and shown in full on page 135)*. The rococo trend of the Aphrodisian school occasionally harks back to Hellenistic prototypes, such as the small 'spinario' group *(bottom)*, yet many other uses of similar genre motifs or groupings - for example the child Herakles strangling the snakes *(below right)* from the Baths of Hadrian - are thoroughly original.

genre scenes or figures, such as the old fisherman. A typically 'rococo' practice is that of placing small figures, or groups, in architectural decorative sculpture, as in the 'peopled scrolls' pilasters — an example is the child Heracles strangling the snakes sent by Hera. Some figural Corinthian revetment capitals display neo-classical tastes within their 'rococo' setting, through the use of well-known statuary types of earlier date, such as the Aphrodite of Cnidus by Praxiteles, or an Apollo with a tripod, placed centrally and framed by the outcurving acanthus leaves of the decoration.

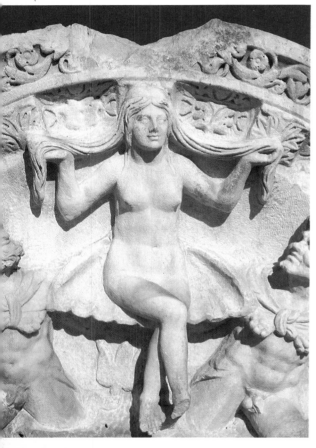

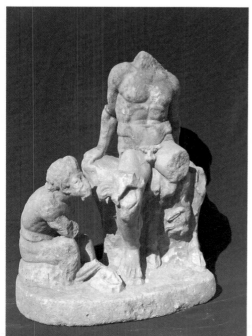

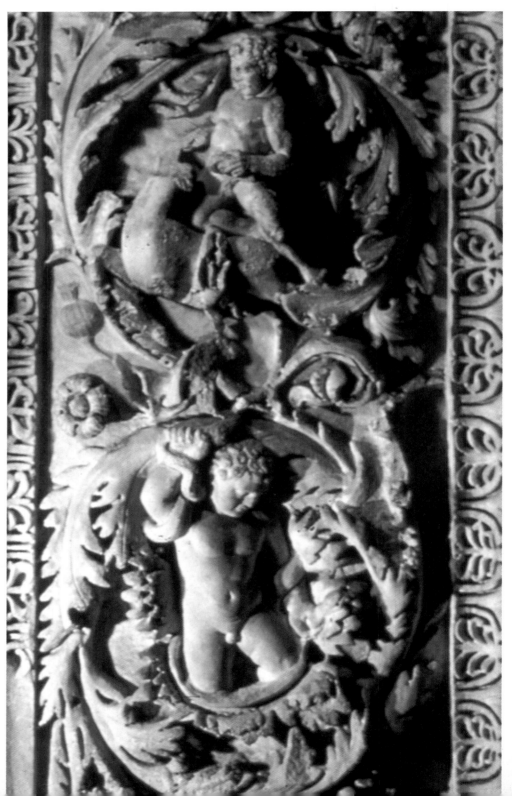

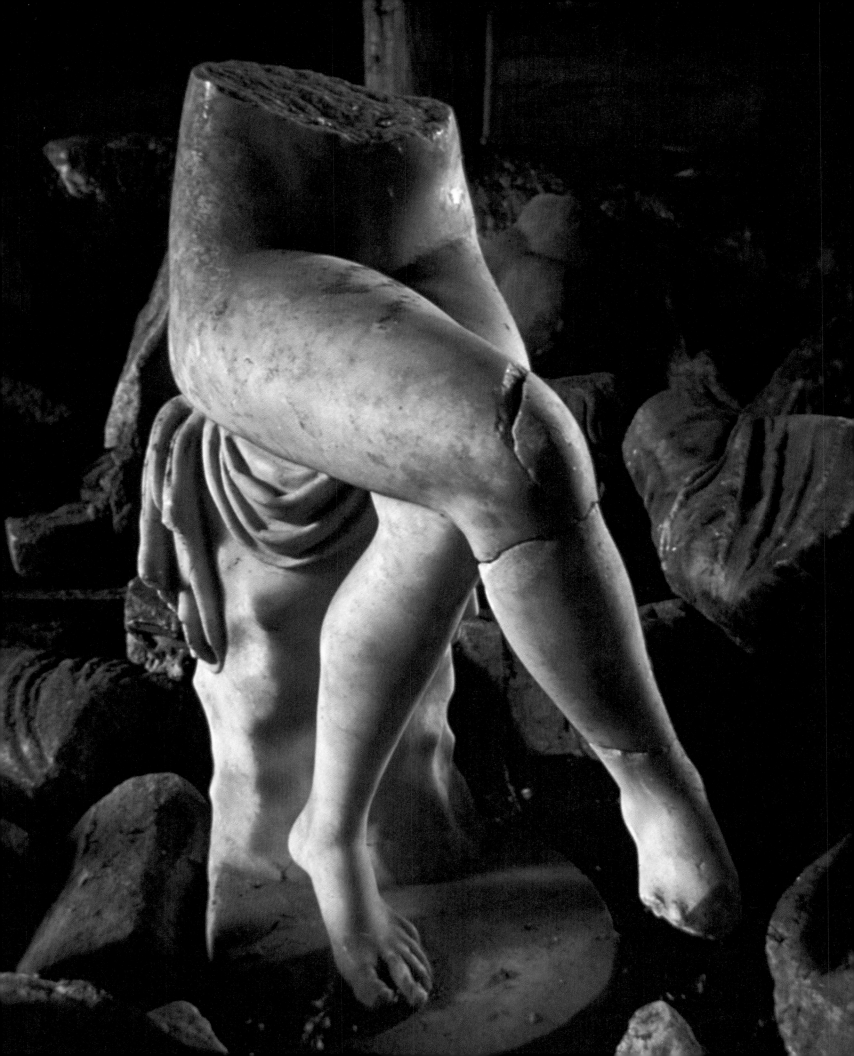

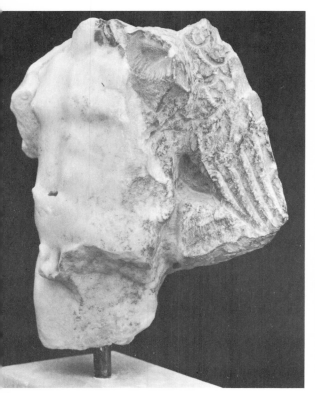

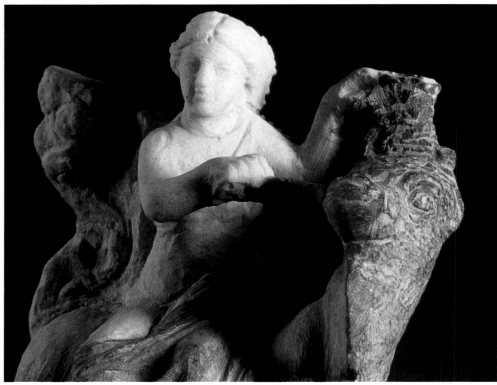

The virtuosity of the Aphrodisian 'school' and its artists' complete mastery over their material are strikingly evident in their carving of bicolour marble pieces, to achieve a cameo-like effect. The white Europa seated on the blue-grey bull *(above right)* and the statuette of Eros *(above)* with blue-grey wings can be considered *tour-de-force* creations.

V. In a similar 'rococo' spirit, the Aphrodisians often used polychromy, sometimes in conjunction with plain white marble. One work of this type is a monumental two-coloured group of a galloping horse, carved out of Aphrodisian blue-grey marble, with a rider carved in white. The two Aphrodisian sculptures of centaurs, now in the Capitoline Museum in Rome, although not examples of polychromy, were carved from a stone of variable grey-black tint referred to as *bigio morato*. There are several specimens of smaller polychrome sculpture that are truly virtuoso pieces. Their sculptors selected naturally two-coloured blocks at the quarries and skilfully carved them to fit the figures of their compositions. In a highly decorative item of this type, showing Europa being abducted by Zeus in the form of a bull, the figure of Europa was so contrived as to be mostly in white, while the lower part of her drapery and the animal remain in blue. A fragmentary statuette of Eros was carved with equal imagination, so that the wings behind the figure are dark blue, while the body is in polished white.

VI. Effects similar to polychromy were achieved in one-colour marble through different finishes of the item's surfaces. The textures of flesh, drapery and hair are distinguished by the soft polishing of one surface to contrast with the rasp-finishing of another, which achieves subtly different effects of light and dark. The seated statue of a poet or philosopher (from the Odeon), where the different textures of the naked torso and the adjacent drapery are cleverly achieved, demonstrates the aesthetic subtlety and technical virtuosity

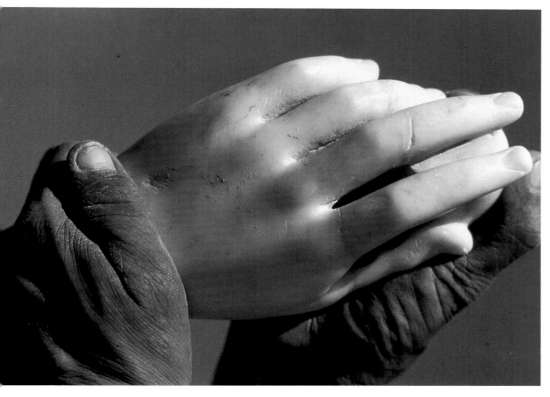

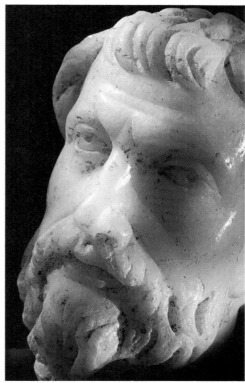

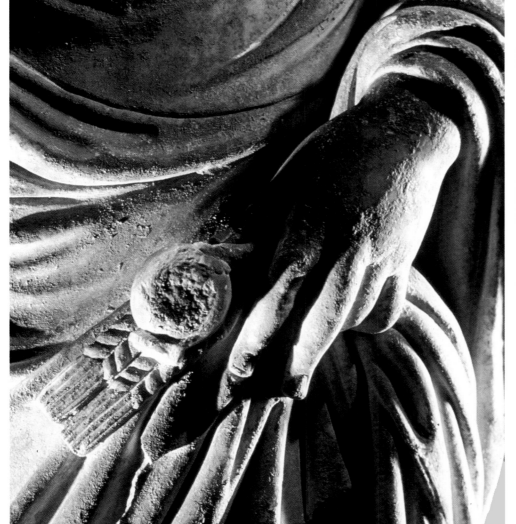

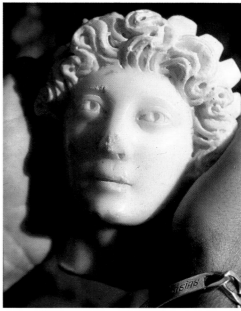

The ability of the Aphrodisians to give extraordinary life to their creations is esspecially evident in their skilful use of different surfaces and finishes in their carvings. It is remarkably evident in the distinct textures of skin, hair and drapery.

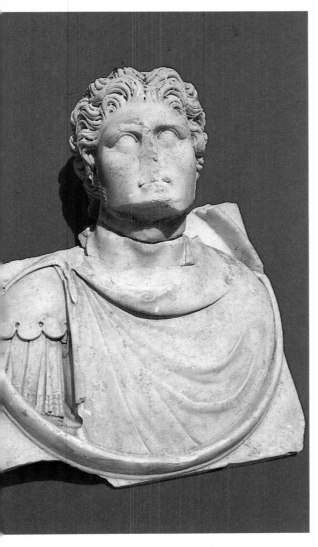

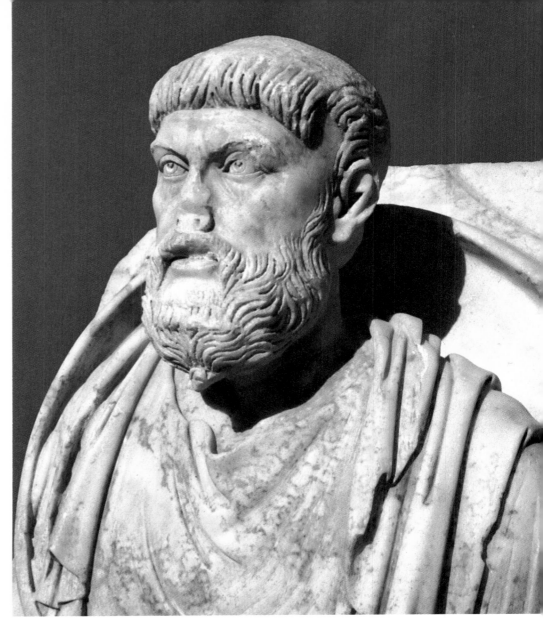

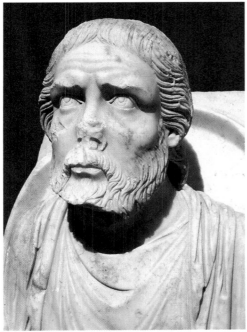

of its sculptor. The same holds true for several portrait heads, among which an exquisitely carved, intact bearded head stands out. Here, the contrast between the highly polished face and the rasp finished hair and beard is further accentuated by the almost translucent, alabaster-like quality of the marble.

VII. A sculpture type not invented by the Aphrodisians, but adopted and adapted by them with great imagination, is the so-called tondo or *imago clipeata* bust. An unusually large number of these decorative portrait busts in circular frames have been found at Aphrodisias, especially in the basilica complex beyond the north portico of the Sebasteion. In these instances, yet again, the Aphrodisians reveal their knowledge of the art of the past. Some of the tondos were inspired by classical portrait types, such as Alcibiades, Pindar, Pythagoras, and Menander. Others, unidentified, are powerful and individual portraits sculpted in late Roman times.

VIII. The most consistent and singularly intriguing characteristic

148

of the Carian sculptors was their unusual technical proficiency. As already noted, the conditions that had generated the 'school', especially the proximity and abundance of marble supplies, were rare enough to permit us to distinguish their technical idiosyncracies and to analyse their development over a period of time, or from one sculptor to another, or between one building and another. A careful study of all the evidence on hand and an examination of the quarries and the quarrying methods used by the Aphrodisians was recently undertaken by Mr Peter Rockwell. His study is probably the first of its kind in the scholarship of ancient sculpture, and his work may provide new insights into the production and technical aspects of ancient sculpture in general, which has been sadly neglected hitherto.

IX. Although the Aphrodisian approach to marble-carving was fairly consistent over the centuries, there were inevitably distinct groups of sculptors or specialists who focused on one particular aspect, depending on their abilities or preferences. Master sculptors undoubtedly executed important commissions of statues in the round. Some were expert portraitists, much in demand by the local gentry. Others distinguished themselves as master craftsmen in carving reliefs. Another group specialized in the execution of architectural sculpture or decoration. Many artists produced small statuary groups for private decorative purposes both at home and abroad. Sarcophagus carving seems to have occupied a great many Aphrodisians, whose contributions to this art form were particularly significant. This can be judged from the vast amount of relevant material recovered in and about Aphrodisias even without a systematic exploration of the city's large necropolis. Judging from the enormous harvest of epigraphy collected at the site in over twenty

Of all ancient sites Aphrodisias has yielded an unprecedented number of tondo busts. Once again, although not an Aphrodisian invention in itself, this type of bust portraiture can be considered to be closely identified with the 'school'. Although often echoing earlier portrait prototypes, the likenesses used in these images became distinctive creations through the typically Aphrodisian skills of character portrayal and interpretation. The three tondos opposite are representative of over a dozen that have been found dating from the third and fourth centuries AD. They show Alexander the Great (top left), the great fifth-century BC poet Pindar, identified by an inscription (top right), and an anonymous thinker or poet (below left).

The sarcophagus production of the Aphrodisian 'school' is another striking feature of marble carving in the Carian region. The contribution of the Aphrodisians to several designs of sarcophagi, such as the garland variety (below), and the columnar or 'Asiatic' type, is quite substantial. This is apparent from current study of the material collected at Aphrodisias, which is already considerable even though no excavations have been conducted in the vast Roman necropolis surrounding the city.

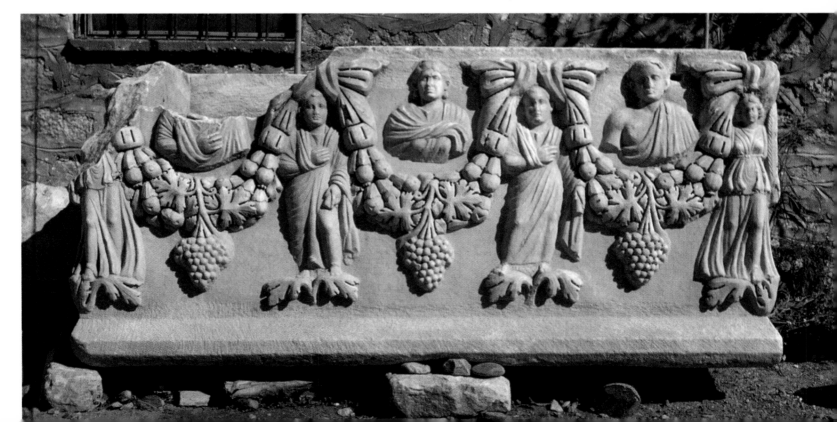

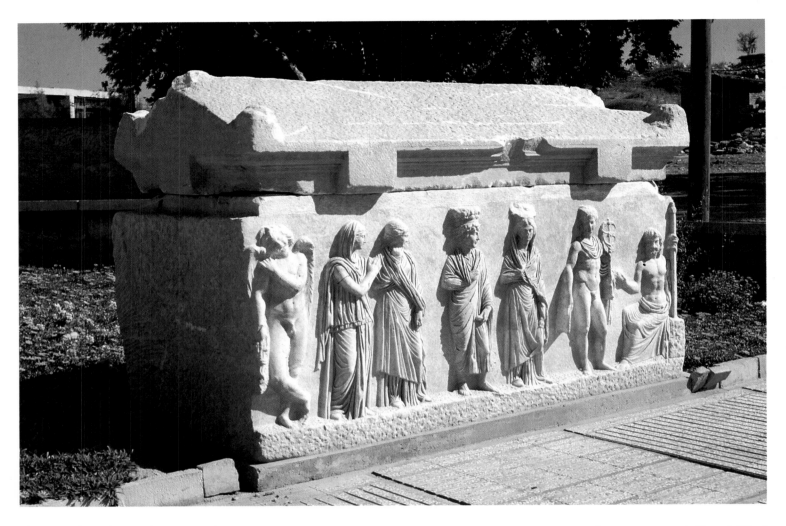

The originality of Aphrodisian sarcophagus designs and their decorations, as well as their techniques of sculpture, are evident in this sarcophagus showing, in the centre, the deceased couple, flanked on their right by Demeter and Persephone and on their left by Hermes Psychopompos. The whole group is framed on one side by *Hypnos* (sleep) or *Thanatos* (death) resting on his elbow and holding a lowered flaming torch and on the other by Hades, who welcomes the couple to his underworld domain.

years, there was even one class of stone-craftsmen especially skilled in the cutting of inscriptions.

It is probable that a definite hierarchy existed among these various groups of artists, craftsmen and their apprentices, and that there were distinctions in the administration and the development of individual workshops. It is premature, however, at the present level of our knowledge, to speculate on such 'distinctions' or to elaborate on the more practical aspects of the 'school': such as the ownership of the quarries, the export production, the economics of the marble trade and the transportation methods and routes.

X.   The regular and continuous training and perfecting of the art of marble-carving among the Aphrodisians are particularly striking. The discovery of the special workshop area clearly illustrates their practices and discrimination. Perhaps even more interesting in this context are the unusual amounts of trial or unfinished pieces that are recovered almost every year during excavations. The inventory of such 'exercise' items, including feet and hands, is fascinating. By their sheer quantity, these should prove beyond reasonable doubt the existence of a highly active 'school' at Aphrodisias.

150

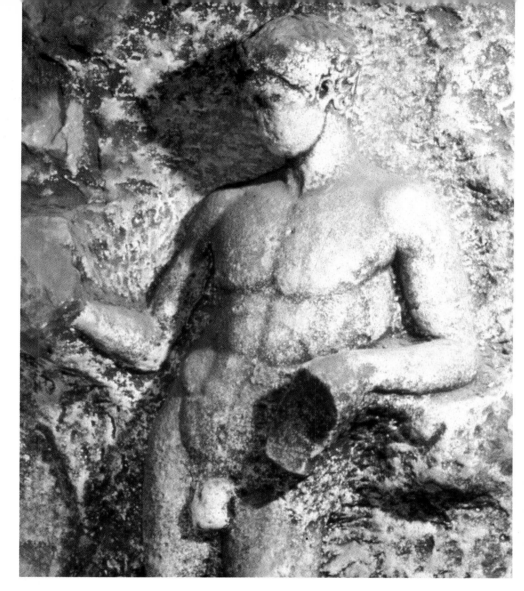

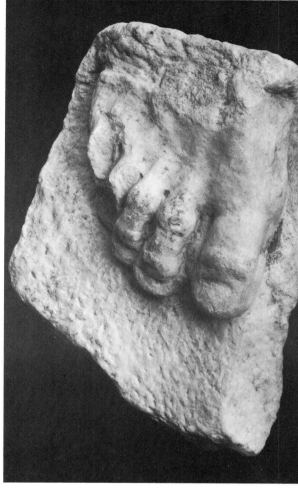

Through these main traits, and others to be refined as the detailed scholarly evaluation of the Aphrodisians proceeds, the character of this 'school' acquires a definite, undeniable individuality. As research continues, we see more and more clearly that the Aphrodisians were an unusual group of artists who succeeded in maintaining a certain homogeneity without loss of individuality and who were always fully aware of the accomplishments of past sculptors. The longevity of the school and the continuous renewal of its vitality from one generation to another, can be explained partly by the proximity of the quarries — which gave Aphrodisian artists an intimate understanding of their material — and partly by their readiness to absorb past examples. They were virtuosi but they were not mere copyists. Analysis of their methods has revealed a loose system of measurement and a reliance on the eye of the individual sculptor that make it clear that they were never simply imitators. They were, rather, inspired interpreters of the past, in the way that a performing musician is the interpreter of a concerto or symphony. Their specific affinities were with Hellenistic sculpture, and particularly that of Pergamon. And so the school can be regarded as the logical, and even the organic, continuation of Pergamene art.

Whatever the reason for the incomplete work on the sarcophagus *(opposite)*, many unfinished sculpture pieces found at Aphrodisias are easily explained because of their association with workshops – either as trial pieces, such as the foot (above) or as work in progress, such as the Hermes *(above left)*. An unprecedented quantity of such unfinished pieces has been recorded in the course of excavations, illustrating the Aphrodisians' emphasis on constant training, practice and perfectionism, which is borne out in the superb quantity of their finished works.

151

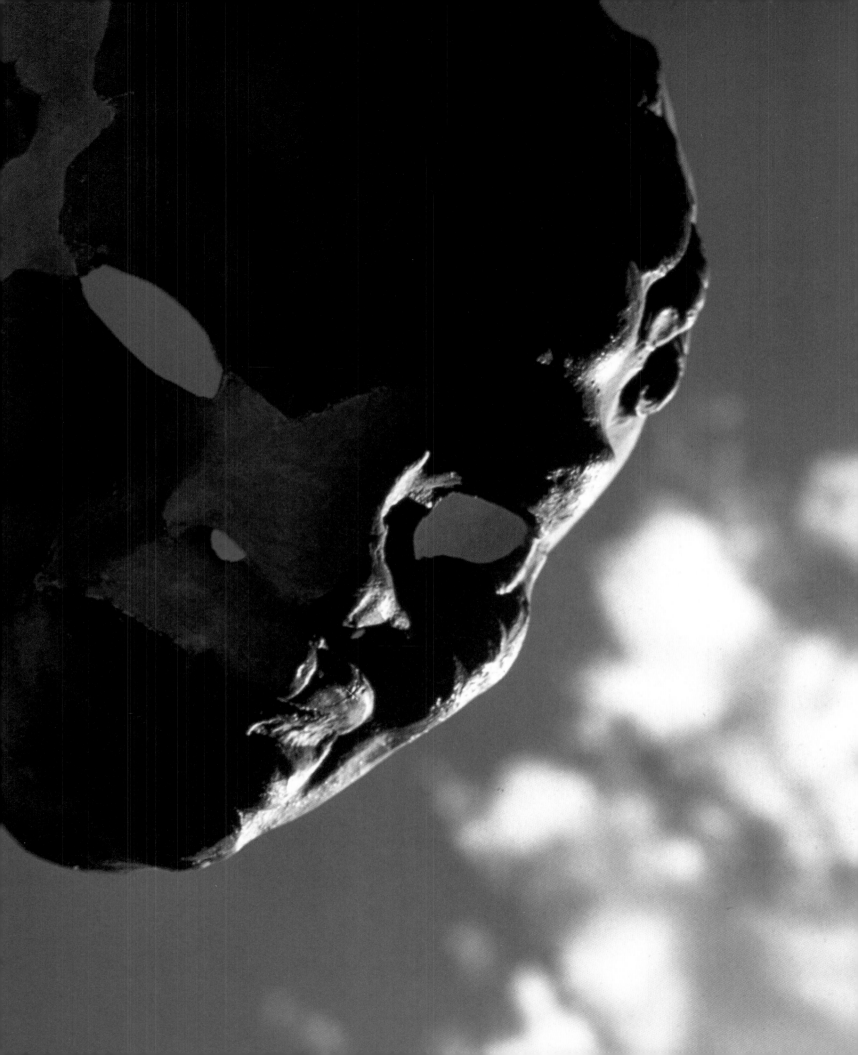

CHAPTER SIX

The Future of Aphrodisias

"In Turkey, a journey without history is like the portrait of an old face without its wrinkles. Every bay or headland of these shores, every mountain top…carries visible or invisible signs of its past. The spell of these landscapes is that their names and stories are familiar, so that one wanders as if through an inherited estate, discovering it anew…"

Freya Stark, *The Lycian Shore*

Freya Stark wrote these lines over thirty years ago. Few have expressed more felicitously the feelings that archaeological sites in Turkey aroused then and still arouse now. Naturally, many changes have taken place since her travels in Asia Minor, some inevitable, some welcome, some perhaps less fortunate. Like ourselves, she experienced Aphrodisias first after a long, laborious journey up from the Maeander valley. Today, that same trip takes about forty minutes by car thanks to a good, well-kept asphalt road built by the Turkish Department of Highways.

Inevitably, after over twenty years of excavation, Aphrodisias no longer consists of only a few clusters of elegant columns lost in the greenery of poplar groves, or ruins silhouetted dramatically against the dark purple mountains, or a huge weed-grown stadium and some occasional, pathetic fortification walls. To regular yearly visitors like ourselves, the extent of changes may at first appear less obvious. However, if Freya Stark, or anyone else, returned to the city of Aphrodite after a lapse of many years, they might at first be startled by the difference between then and now, but they would soon come to appreciate the equilibrium that has been preserved between past and present.

Of course, the old village of Geyre, with its tottering stone cottages that stood over the ancient city, has in great part disappeared. A few of its more typical houses, however, have been, or will be, restored and preserved as testimony to this more recent phase of Aphrodisias' history.

Beneath the old stone cottages and the dusty alley-ways, however, evidence of a more glorious past has emerged and more is still coming, to light. The Museum now graces one side of what was

A terracota mask of a negroid face found near the Odeon stands dramatically against the clear blue Aphrodisian sky.

153

once the village square, but the magnificent plane tree and the two ancient marble seats dragged under its shade by some unknown villager have remained untouched. The former coffee-house nearby and its adjacent stables with their wooden posts standing on ancient column bases have been consolidated. The graceful poplar groves that resemble lovely plumes against the sky still sway in the summer breeze. Farmers still grow corn, other cereal, melon or grape crops in neighbouring fields. Clusters of pomegranate bushes and fragrant fig and apple trees continue to pour forth their fruits to the delight of increasingly frequent busloads of visitors. Limpid waters still run over the moss-covered column drums of the Agora to the accompaniment of the monotonous cooing of turtle doves by day or the croaking of frogs by night.

Thus, despite unavoidable changes, the unique atmosphere and gem-like setting of Aphrodisias have been maintained. For our yearly archaeological labours have been directed almost as much toward safeguarding the site's extraordinary charm as to unravelling its unusually rich past through the study of the varied and abundant archaeological material unearthed.

Much of our work today concentrates on research and the interpretation of our rich harvest of archaeological finds, whether sculpture, inscriptions, architecture, pottery, mosaics, coins, glass, terracottas, jewellery or utilitarian objects. In due course, this will culminate in a series of scholarly volumes presenting the results of our investigations to the academic community and the public at large. Already two such studies, one focusing on a group of significant inscriptions and the other on our rich prehistoric finds, extol the name of the site. Other dedicated collaborators are still pursuing their painstaking and definitive studies.

Aphrodisias has not yet, however, yielded all the secrets that lie concealed in its rich soil. There are still exciting discoveries to be

Although sculpture finds have provided the richest vein at Aphrodisias, an equally impressive quantity of pottery, small artefacts of all types and coins have been recovered over the past twenty-five years. Among these, some of the most interesting include late Roman and Byzantine bronze spoons *(below right)* a Byzantine silver brooch *(below)* and a bronze reliquary cross *(opposite page)*. Both the brooch and the cross were found in Byzantine tombs which were often encountered in the course of excavations within the walls. In contrast to earlier extramural burial practices, Christian burials were allowed within the city walls.

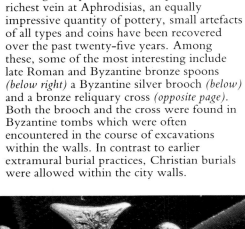

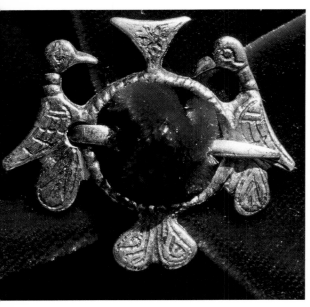

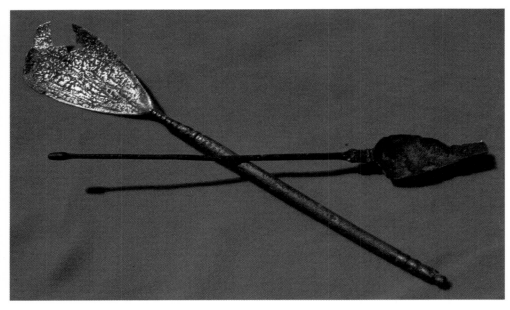

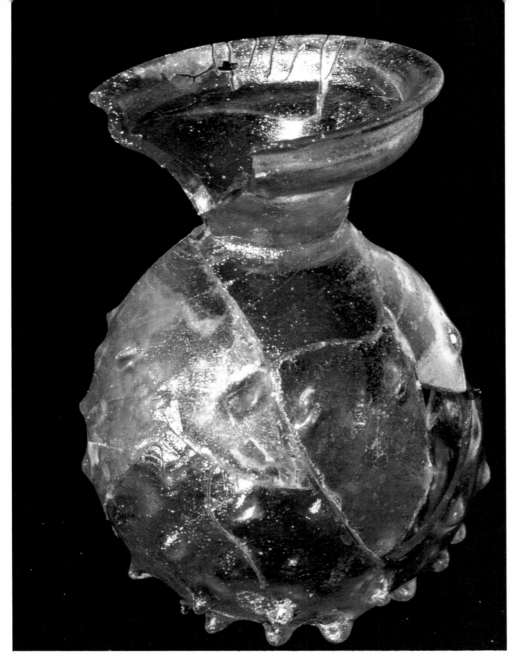

Although fragile and delicate, some late Roman and Byzantine glass vessels have been miraculously preserved. Among them, one of the most beautiful, is this small perfume bottle *(left)*.

A huge collection of Greek, Roman and Byzantine coins collected from various locations within the city – and added to constantly by the gifts of other similar coins found nearby by local workmen and villagers – continues to be a source for important studies soon to be published.

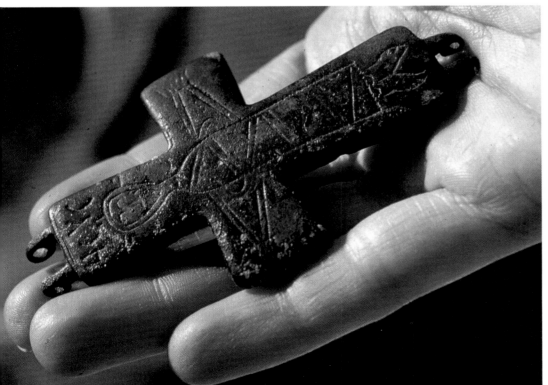

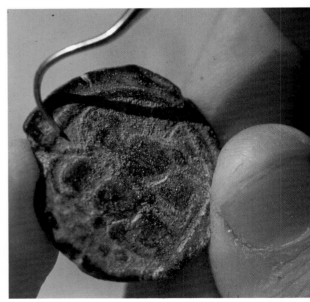

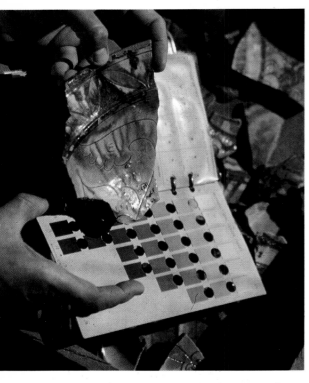

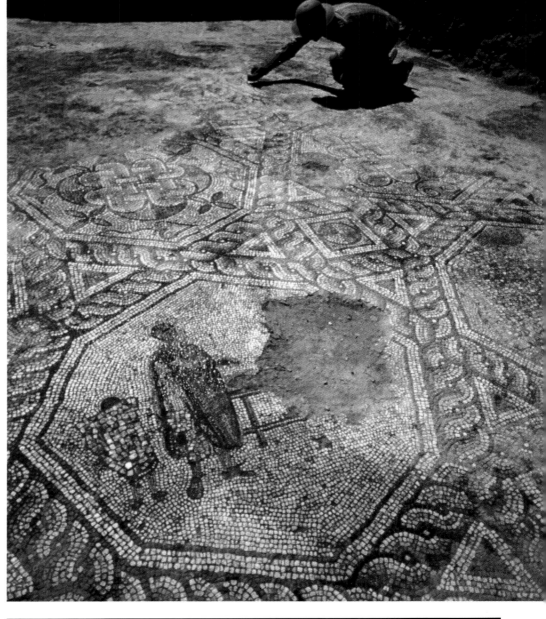

Almost from the very beginning of the project, but at a more accelerated pace in recent years, the preservation, protection, conservation, restoration and study of the finds at Aphrodisias have been major priorities. Some mosaics such as one found near the south wall of the city *(opposite right)* have been consolidated for their protection and reburied for future study. Bronze Age *(below left)* as well as Byzantine pottery *(above)* continue to be studied and restored, while inscriptions *(below right)* provide additional crucial information about the history of the site.

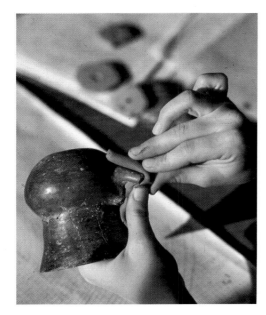

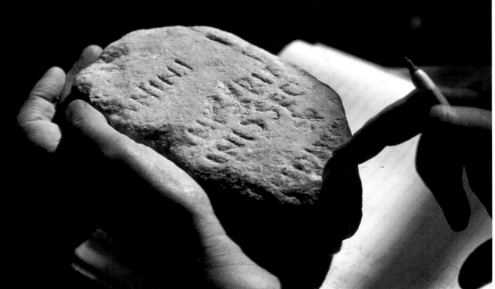

156

made and important developments to be witnessed. Barely twenty per cent of the ancient site has been probed by our spades. For example, the precise plan and development of the city remains unclear, and, out of necessity, only a few private dwellings have been investigated. Those that have been excavated have been found to be decorated with handsome mosaics on their floors and frescoes on their walls. Furthermore, the agora and the huge Roman necropolis stretching in all directions beyond the fortification walls have yet to be fully explored.

Almost all the collection of sarcophagi in and around the Museum either stem from the Gaudin excavations of 1904–1905 or were found and reused by villagers in or near Geyre. Some were recovered in the course of recent salvage operations, but there are only a few of these because burial was not permitted within the city limits in classical times, except for a limited number of special individuals. With the advent of Christianity, however, burials *intra muros* became usual, particularly in association with churches, chapels or other consecrated ground. Many such tombs were encountered and excavated in the course of our operations, above all in the proximity of the cathedral of the Byzantine city, which had formerly been the Temple of Aphrodite.

The continued presence of Geyre and its network of roads and alleys often thwarted exploration of the public or private building complexes we had discovered. These excavations are occasionally resumed as our schedule and funds allow, since they are essential to the interpretation of monuments such as the Sebasteion and the Tetrapylon.

As well as excavation, even more delicate and challenging duties confront us. Foremost among these are the protection, preservation and careful, unobtrusive restoration of the remains and works of art that we have already uncovered. Fortunately, with the assistance and

Restoration of pottery involves the completion of many important vessels by plaster replacement of missing fragments. An unusual late seventh-century BC vessel is shown *(below left)* being repaired by Reha Arican in the laboratory of the Museum. In addition to examination of actual fragments, the study inscriptions – particularly on larger stones, of which there is an abundance at Aphrodisias – requires not only good photographs to be taken but also 'squeezes' to be made either with specially wetted paper or with liquid rubber compound. The last procedure is shown being carried out by the author.

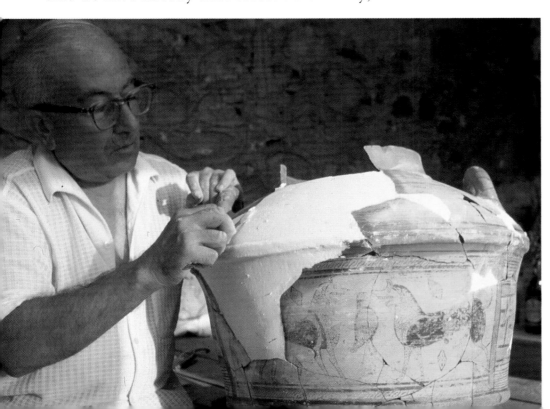

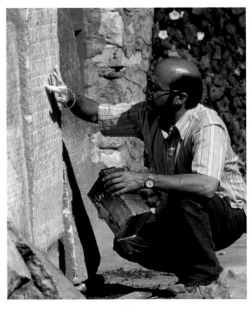

A more costly and difficult responsibility of the archaeologist is the preservation and protection of large-scale monumental remains uncovered by excavation. This has been readily assumed, although with limited financial and mechanical means, by the Aphrodisias project. A considerable amount of unobtrusive repair, consolidation and re-erection of columns has been achieved so far and continues. One of the most satisfactory achievements of this type is the restoration programme of the basilica-type hall in the Theatre Baths, which contains two rows of beautiful columns of local blue-grey marble *(below)* and square posts and 'peopled scrolls' pillars, shown in the process of re-erection *(opposite page)*.

co-operation of the Directorate-General of Antiquities and Museums of Turkey, and support from the National Geographic Society, several important initial steps toward fulfilling these obligations have been taken. The Museum has been built and the removal of old Geyre through expropriation has been greatly accelerated . . . yet safeguarding Aphrodisias as a complete archaeological complex remains a vital issue.

The official measures taken in 1976 by the Turkish High Commission for Monuments, Yüksek Anıtlar Kurulu (subsequently reorganised, this commission now bears the name Taşinmaz Kültür ve Tabiat Varlıkları Yüksek Kurulu, the High Commission for Permanent Cultural and Natural Resources), and the acceleration of expropriations in key areas of the site, have already been alluded to. However picturesque village life may appear against the background of ancient remains, sadly it hinders the protection and restoration of these monuments. Furthermore, the possibility of unsuitable development in the vicinity of the site for purposes of tourism must not be discounted.

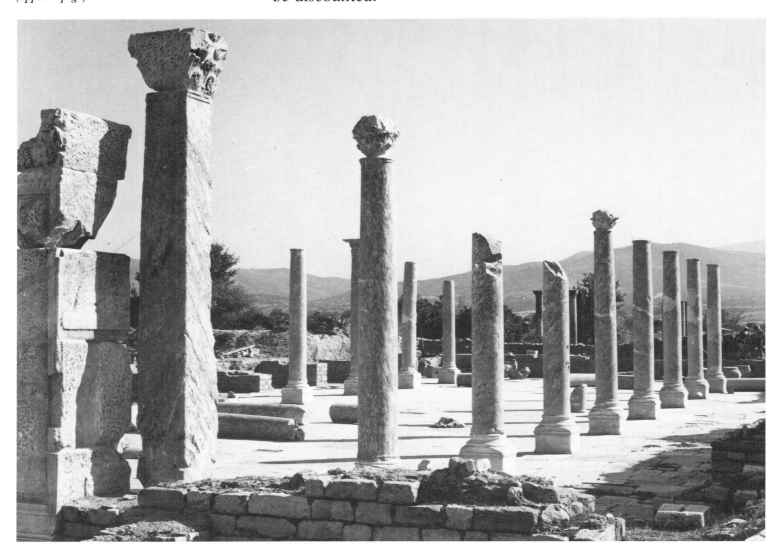

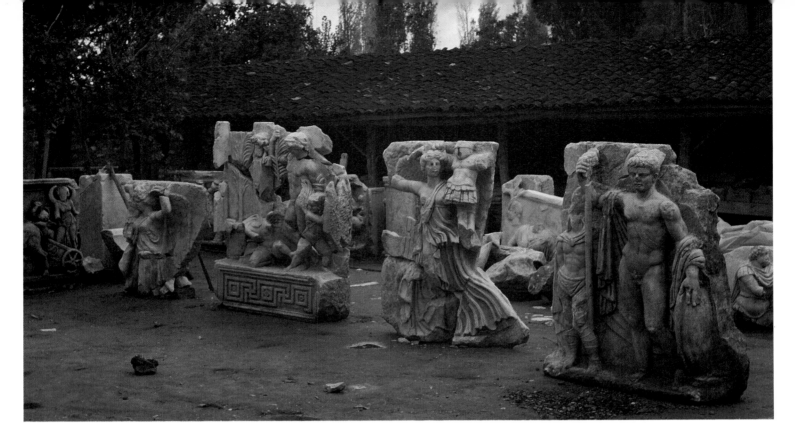

A more sensitive problem facing the project is the huge collection of all kinds of monumental and decorative sculpture discovered since the completion of the Aphrodisias Museum. For their protection, and because of the lack of storage space in the Museum, these are currently safeguarded within the compound of the excavation headquarters. The long-term future of this superb collection and of all the extraordinarily rich remains at Aphrodisias ultimately depends on the creation of an archaeological park, which will not only allow excavation and study to continue unhindered but will also permit this beautiful, unplundered and unique site to be fully appreciated by the public at large.

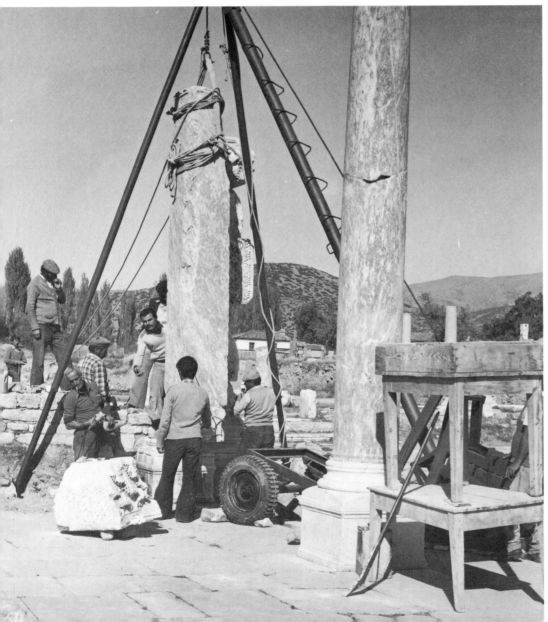

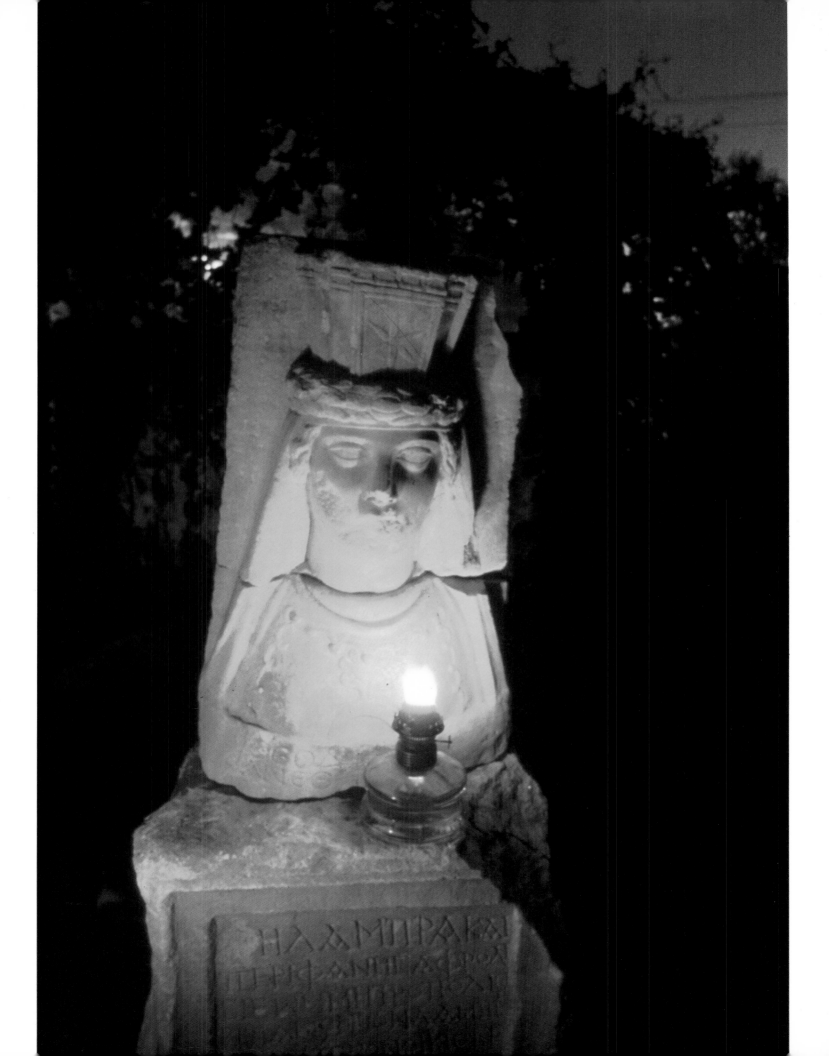

The acquisition of the whole site as defined in 1976 and the conversion of Aphrodisias into an archaeological park or reservation is a paramount priority. In the interests of the future of the site it must be completed as soon as possible. This will not only safeguard the site for future generations of archaeologists and visitors but will also do much to protect it from unattractive developments.

The inadequate facilities of the present Museum must also be improved. Additional exhibition and storage space is urgently needed for the large number of finds made even before the Museum was completed. Meanwhile, we were obliged to store many sculptures and architectural fragments in the Museum grounds or in the courtyard and gardens of our excavation headquarters nearby. Also, the modest restoration and consolidation work currently being undertaken on several important excavated monuments should be intensified and even extended.

Much effort, dedication and patient perseverance will be required to bring these hopes to fruition in forthcoming years. In many respects, our work relating to such long-term issues, involving as it must so much administration, negotiation and above all fund-raising, is even more arduous than the more directly archaeological aspects of our operations over the past twenty-five years. Despite the now recognized significance of Aphrodisias and the tremendous visual and historical impact of our discoveries, there is still indifference — or even resistance — from those who do not understand or appreciate the validity of preserving history.

Aphrodisias is unique not only as a treasure house of archaeological finds, but also as a place where those willing to establish a dialogue with the past may commune — like the humanists and artists of the great cities of the Italian Renaissance — with the beauty and harmony of the ancient world. In few places is this so evident as here. It must be preserved at all costs. One must hope and trust that the many visitors to the site, and the readers of this book who have not had the opportunity to visit Aphrodisias, will grasp the feelings that impel us so strongly to protect and preserve the extraordinary beauty of its past.

After centuries of prosperity and decline, the patron goddess of the site and the city - the Aphrodite of Aphrodisias - still watches over her sacred realm.

161

Chronological Table

PREHISTORIC PERIOD AT APHRODISIAS (Dates are approximate)	
c. 5800 BC	Late Neolithic (New Stone) Age (?)
c. 5300–4360 BC	
c. 4360–2915 BC	Late Chalcolithic (Copper Stone) Age
c. 2915–2800 BC	Late Chalcolithic–Early Bronze Age I
c. 2800–2600 BC	
c. 2600–2500 BC	Early Bronze Age 2
c. 2500–2400 BC	Early Bronze Age 3
c. 2400–2300/2200 BC	Early Bronze Age 4
c. 2300/2200–1900 BC	Early Bronze Age 4 – Middle Bronze Age
c. 1900–(?)1600 BC	Middle Bronze Age Gap
c. 1600–(?)1300 BC	
c. 1300–1200 BC	Late Bronze Age
from c. 1200–1100 (?) BC	Iron Age

ARCHAIC PERIOD c. 680–480 BC		
c. 680–546 BC	West Asia Minor becomes part of Persian Empire	"Lydian" period at Aphrodisias
After 546 BC		
Later sixth century BC		Evidence of cult of "Aphrodite" at Aphrodisias, probably with a temple.
	Founding of Roman Republic	
509 BC	Persian Wars	
493–479 BC		

CLASSICAL PERIOD 480–400 BC

431–404 BC	Golden Age of Athens Athenian Empire Peloponnesian War	

FOURTH CENTURY BC

377–353 BC	Mausolus, satrap of Caria	
382–336 BC 336–323 BC	Rise of Macedonian power: Philip II Alexander III (the Great) Alexander conquers the Persian Empire and beyond	

HELLENISTIC PERIOD 323–31 BC

282–133 BC	Alexander's empire divided into three main kingdoms (Antigonid in Greece and Macedonia, Ptolemaic in Egypt and Seleucid in Syria and Mesopotamia) In West Asia Minor, kingdom of Pergamon under the Attalids	The historian, Apollonius of Aphrodisias, writes a history of Caria.
From late third century BC	Rome becomes involved in the Eastern Mediterranean against the Hellenistic monarchies	
189 BC	Battle of Magnesia: defeat of Antiochus III of Syria by Rome	
188 BC	Peace of Apamaea settles in Rome's favour	
133 BC	Death of Attalus III of Pergamon and bequest of his kingdom to Rome After crushing a revolt, Rome creates the province of Asia	Union of Plarasa and Aphrodisias. Treaty of the two with neighbouring Cibyra and Tabae under protection of Rome.
100–90 BC		Links between Plarasa/Aphrodisias and kingdom of Bithynia.
88 BC	First Mithradatic War: Mithradates, King of Pontus, invades province of Asia	Aphrodisias supports Rome.

87 BC	Roman general Sulla fights Mithradates	Sulla advised by Greek oracle to make offerings to Aphrodite of Aphrodisias.
85 BC	Mithradates defeated. Sulla reorganizes Asian cities	Sulla makes his offerings to Aphrodite, perhaps gives her city certain privileges.
83–82 BC	Second Mithradatic War	
78–75 BC	Roman campaigns in Lycia, Pamphylia	Coins issued under the name of Plarasa/Aphrodisias (mostly bronze).
74–63 BC	Third Mithradatic War	
60 BC	First Triumvirate (Pompey, Julius Caesar, Crassus)	
47 BC		Julius Caesar campaigns against Pharnaces, King of Pontus, makes donations to Aphrodite of Aphrodisias; he subsequently grants her sacred precinct rights of asylum.
44 BC	Assassination of Caesar	
43 BC	Second Triumvirate (Antony, Octavian, Lepidus) Brutus and Cassius control Asia Minor and maltreat Caesar's friends	
42 BC	Battle of Philippi: Brutus and Cassius defeated by Antony and Octavian Antony in Asia Minor, helps cities that had suffered under Brutus and Cassius	
40 BC	War against Labienus	With Parthian troops, Labienus invades Asia Minor. Aphrodisias is sacked.
39 BC	Brundisium Pact: Antony and Octavian divide the Mediterranean into spheres of influence.	Octavian asserts a patron's rights over Aphrodisias, essentially in Antony's territory. Decree and law sponsored by both triumvirs passed at Rome conferring privileges on Aphrodisias. Loot taken by Labienus and his men recovered thanks to Octavian's intervention.

164

39 BC		C. Julius Zoilos, Octavian's freeman, involved in the delimitation of an extended area of asylum in the precinct of Aphrodite. Building or rebuilding programme, especially the Temple of Aphrodite, the Theatre and the agora.

ROMAN PERIOD

31 BC	Battle of Actium	
30 BC	Defeat and deaths of Antony and Cleopatra Octavian, sole ruler	
27 BC	Octavian becomes Augustus	Building activities continue at Aphrodisias; cult in honour of Augustus initiated.
	Augustus, Agrippa (his son-in-law) and his adopted son Gaius visit Asia Minor	
AD 14	Death of Augustus Tiberius emperor	Continued building programme at Aphrodisias in agora (Portico of Tiberius) and Sebasteion with extension of cult of the Imperial house.
17	Major earthquake in Asia Minor	Aphrodisias damaged.
17-19	Germanicus, Tiberius' adopted son visits Asia Minor.	Sculptor Koblanos active in Italy
22		Confirmation of asylum rights by Tiberius
37	Death of Tiberius	
37-41	Gaius (Caligula) emperor	
41-54	Claudius emperor	Extension and reorganization of cult of imperial family at Aphrodisias.
c. 47	Earthquake in Asia Minor	Aphrodisias damaged.
54	Death of Claudius	
54-68	Nero emperor	

55–60 and 62–66	Campaigns in Armenia	Victories illustrated in Sebasteion at Aphrodisias.
68	Crisis: Year of Four Emperors	
69	Accession of Vespasian and Flavian Dynasty	Chariton, writer of romance *Chaereas and Callirhoe* hails from Aphrodisias.
79	Death of Vespasian	Xenocrates, medical writer, active at Aphrodisias.
79–81	Titus emperor	
81–96	Domitian emperor	Construction of aqueducts at Aphrodisias. Aphrodisias contributes to offering made in honour of Domitian at Ephesus.
96–98	Nerva emperor	Sculptor Zenon, son of Attinas.
98–117	Trajan emperor	Privileges of Aphrodisias upheld according to surviving letter.
between 102–116		Earthquake causes damage at Aphrodisias.
101–2 and 105–6	Dacian Wars	Sculptor Apollonius
117–138	Hadrian emperor	Privileges of Aphrodisias upheld according to surviving letter.
		Large bath building erected at Aphrodisias.
		Sculptors, Antoninos, Aristeas and Papias from Aphrodisias active at Rome. Also P. Likinios Priskos, Zenion and Zenon, son of Alexander active elsewhere.
138–161	Accession of Antoninus Pius and Antonine Dynasty	Adrastos, peripatetic philosopher, hails from Aphrodisias.
161–180	Marcus Aurelius emperor (till 169, with Lucius Verus)	
162–166	Parthian Wars	
180–192	Commodus emperor	Privileges of Aphrodisias upheld according to surviving letter. Official appointed to assist in

		organization of funds for financing games and musical competitions.
192	Crisis: Series of civil wars, involving Asia Minor	
192-211	Accession of Septimius Severus and Severan Dynasty	
198	Caracalla, eldest son, becomes joint emperor with Severus	Alexander, peripatetic philosopher hailing from Aphrodisias, lectures on Aristotle at Athens, and dedicates one of his books to Septimius Severus and Caracalla.
		Privileges of Aphrodisias upheld according to surviving epigraphical documents.
		Several Aphrodisians attested as senators at Rome. Sculptor Alexander, son of Zenon.
211	Caracalla and brother Geta emperors	
212	*Constitutio Antoniniana* confers citizenship on all free men	
212	Murder of Geta	
215-216	Caracalla and Julia Domna travel in Asia Minor	
217	Death of Caracalla	
217-218	Macrinus emperor	
218-222	Elagabalus emperor	
222-235	Alexander Severus emperor	Privileges of Aphrodisias upheld according to surviving letter.
235-238	Maximinus Thrax emperor	
238	Gordian I, then Gordian II emperors	Sculptor Polyneikes
238-244	Gordian III emperor	Privileges of Aphrodisias upheld according to several letters.
242-243	Wars against Persia	
244-249	Philip (the Arab) emperor	

249-251	Traianus Decius emperor	Privileges of Aphrodisias upheld according to surviving epigraphical document.
251-253	Trebonianus Gallus emperor	
253	Crisis: Several claimants to throne, soon superseded by Valerian, who is associated with his son Gallienus.	New province organized at this time joining Caria and Phrygia, probably with Aphrodisias as its capital.
260	Parthian Wars: Valerian captured.	
260-268	Gallienus emperor	
268-270	Claudius II Gothicus emperor	
270-275	Aurelian emperor	
275-276	Tacitus emperor	
276-282	Probus emperor	
282-283	Carus emperor	
283-284	Numerian emperor	
283-285	Carinus emperor	
284-305	Diocletian emperor: Establishment of Tetrarchy with reorganisation of empire: Diocletian and Maximianus as co-Augusti; Galerius and Constantius as co-Caesars	
301	*Edict of Maximum Prices* and revaluation of currency promulgated	Both edicts set up on panels at Aphrodisias near a reorganized large basilica off the agora.
301-305		Caria becomes a separate province with Aphrodisias as its capital.
306-312	Maxentius emperor	
308-324	Licinius emperor	

BYZANTINE PERIOD

307–337	Accession of Constantine I (the Great) as sole ruler; establishment of Constantinian dynasty	
324		
313	Edict of Milan: End of Christian persecutions	
325	Council of Nicaea: Christianity becomes the religion of the Empire	Ammonius, first bishop of Aphrodisias attends the Council.
326	New capital established at Byzantium, now renamed Constantinople.	
337–361	Constantius II emperor	
c. 359		Building of west (or Antioch) gate of fortification system.
359		Serious earthquake causes much damage in western Asia Minor, and at Aphrodisias.
361–363	Julian the Apostate emperor. Attempts at pagan revival	Antonius Tatianus, governor of Caria, builds the Tetrastoon, to the east of the Theatre
360s		Completion of city wall system.
379–395	Accession of Theodosius I (the Great) and the Theodosian dynasty	
395–408	Arcadius emperor	
408–450	Theodosius II emperor	
431	Council of Ephesus	Cyrus, bishop of Aphrodisias, attends.
443		Theodosius II visits Aphrodisias
		Temple of Aphrodite probably converted to a basilica at this time.
449	Council of Ephesus ("Robber Synod") recognizes monophysite doctrine	Cyrus attends.
	Council of Chalcedon	Critonianus, bishop of Aphrodisias, attends.

450s		Remodelling and transformation of Agora Gate into a *nymphaeum*. Repairs to city walls, and Odeon.
455	Sack of Rome by Vandals	
457–474	Accession of Leo I and his dynasty	
480s		Asklepiodotos of Alexandria, a Neoplatonist philosopher, takes up residence at Aphrodisias. Paganism, as well as monophysite christianity, in the city.
474–491	Zenon emperor	
491–518	Anastasius emperor	
Late fifth century		Flavius Palmatus, governor of Caria and acting "vicar" of Asia honoured at Aphrodisias with erection of a statue.
518–527	Dynasty of Justinian: Justin I emperor	
518		Euphemius, bishop of Aphrodisias, exiled for monophysite activities.
527–565	Justinian I (the Great) emperor	
c. 529		Aphrodisians petition emperor to protect interest payments that they receive from their endowments.
565–578	Justin II emperor	
582–602	Maurice Tiberius emperor	
602–610	Usurper Phocas emperor	
610–641	Accession of Heraclius and his dynasty	
Early seventh century		Major earthquake brings much damage to Aphrodisias. Little repair is attempted. Spolia used to create a citadel on the 'acropolis' over ruins of Theatre. Change of name of the city to Stavropolis.
611–627	Persians invade Anatolia	
632	Rise of Islam	

635–641	Arab conquests in Middle East	
	Arabs attack Constantinople	
685–695 and 705–711	Justinian II emperor	
717–741	Accession of Leo III and Isaurian dynasty	
717–718	Arab siege of Constantinople	
726	Beginning of Iconoclast Controversy	
741–775	Constantine V Copronymus emperor	
775–780	Leo IV the Khazar	
787	Council of Nicaea: Condemnation of Iconoclasm	
843	Final restoration of Images	
876–912	Accession of Basil I and Macedonian dynasty	
886–912	Leo VI emperor	
913–959	Constantine VII Porphyrogenitus emperor	
959–963	Romanus II emperor	
963–969 969–976	Usurpers Nicephorus II Phocas and John I Zimisces	
976–1025	Accession of Basil II Bulgarochtonos and his Macedonian dynasty	In tenth or eleventh century, repairs and alterations in main church, or cathedral, of Aphrodisias (ex-temple of Aphrodite).
1054	Separation of Greek and Roman Churches	
1057–1078	Dynasty of Dukas and Comnenes	
1064	Seljuk Turks in eastern Anatolia	
1071	Battle of Manzikert: defeat of Byzantine armies	
1078	Seljuk Turks in western Asia Minor	

ISLAMIC PERIOD

1081–1181	Accession of Alexius I Comnenus and Comnene dynasty	Aphrodisias (alias Caria) attacked by Seljuk Turks.
1143–1180	Manuel I emperor	
1147–1149	The Second Crusade	
1188		Theodore Mangaphas, in rebellion against emperor, sacks Caria with Seljuk raiders.
1189–1192	The Third Crusade	
1195–1203	Alexius III emperor	Sultan of Iconium (Konya) seizes Caria. 5,000 people captured and resettled at Philomelium.
1201–1204	The Fourth Crusade Capture and sack of Constantinople in 1204	
1204–1261	Latin empire of Constantinople	
1204–1261	Byzantine emperors of Nicaea	
1261–1282	Accession of Michael VIII Palaeologus and dynasty of Palaeologi	Brief revival of Byzantine rule in Maeander valley.
c. 1279		Caria once again seized by Seljuk and Turcoman raiders. Remaining population resettled elsewhere.
1308	The Ottoman Turks in western Asia Minor and Europe	
1328–1341	Andronicus III emperor	By end of fourteenth century Caria (alias Aphrodisias) ceases to be mentioned in the lists of sees.
1449–1453	Constantine XI Dragases emperor	
1453	Siege and capture of Constantinople by Mehmet II and the Turks	

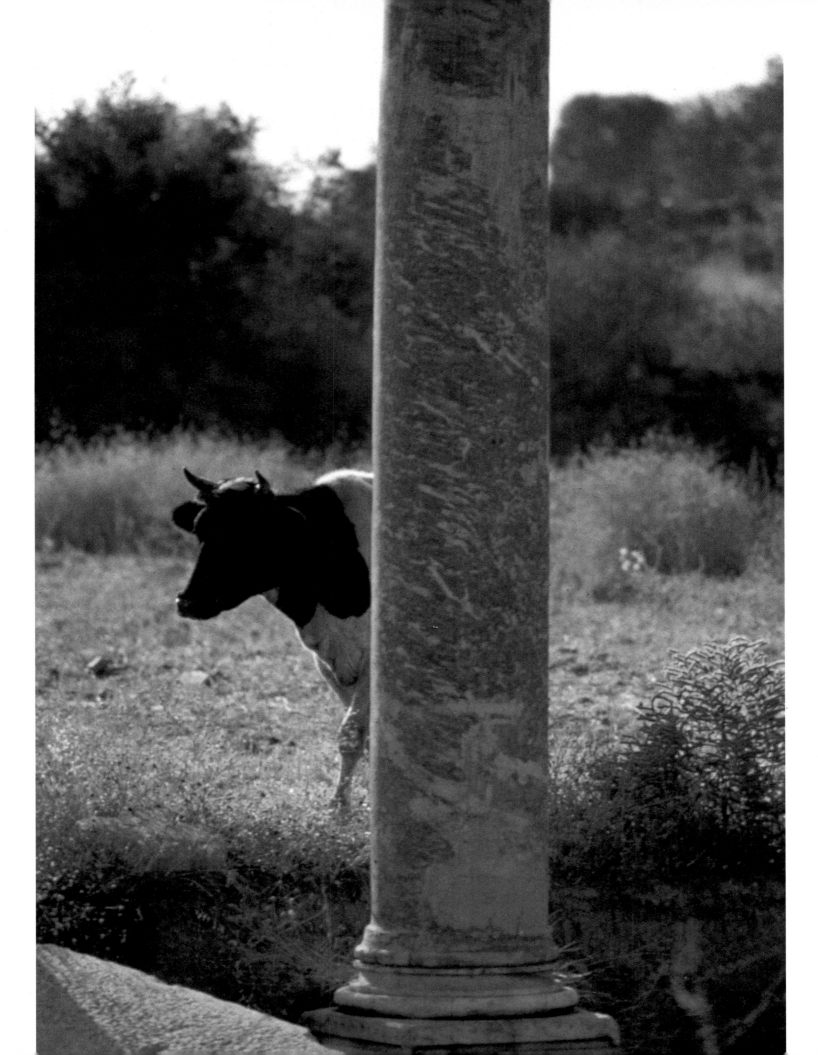

Select Glossary

As with all similar glossaries, the one which follows cannot pretend to be exhaustive. However, it attempts to include most of the words, expressions or terms that may not be familiar to all readers. Some Greek terms are given in their original transcribed forms, especially when they are epigraphically attested to. Many are in a commonly used Latin or English form. Classical plurals are added, where relevant. For ancient geographical names, the reader is advised to consult the maps on pages 16–17 and 32–33 of this book.

acropolis (lit. 'high city') Citadel, or fortified height of an ancient Greek city.

acroterium(-a) Ornamental Finial(s) placed at angles; including the apex of a pediment.

aedicula(-ae) Diminutive of (Lat.) *aedes* = temple, used to refer to columnar units or niches, or pilastered tabernacles. Frequently encountered in elaborate ornamental façades (hence adj. 'aediculated') of theatre stages, gateways, fountain-houses or similar constructions of the Graeco-Roman period.

agora Market-place or area of an ancient Greek city. (Roman equivalent: *forum*).

Amazon Mythological nation or people of female warriors usually located on the fringes of the ancient world, according to Greek tradition, and connected with several legends, myths or heroes (e.g. Trojan War, Heracles, Theseus, etc.). Amazons are very frequently represented in classical art fighting Greeks, hence the term 'Amazonomachy' (lit. 'Amazon fight') applied to such combat scenes.

analemma(-ata) Walls sustaining the forward projecting ends of the *cavea* (or auditorium) of a Greek theatre.

Anatolia Essentially modern geographic term used for the Asiatic portion of Turkey.

anta(-ae) Wall ends, or pilasters at the extremities of the side walls of the *cella* of a temple. When columns are placed in the façade between these two ends or pilasters, they are said to be *in antis*.

174

antefix   Decorative element placed at the ends of rows of cover tiles of a roof in order to conceal the joints of the flat tiles.

apodyterium   Dressing, or changing room, in a Roman bath.

archaic   Adjective used conventionally in connection with the art and architecture of the pre-classical period, i.e. from the seventh century to c. 500 BC.

Asia   In a Roman historical context, a province formed out of the territory of the kingdom of Pergamon bequeathed in 133 BC to Rome by Attalus III, and including most of western Anatolia. Originally consisted of the ancient regions of Mysia, Lydia, Ionia, Caria, and eventually (after 116) Phrygia.

atrium   Central hall of a Roman private house. In an early Byzantine or Christian church, the word refers to a front court, usually framed by four porticoes or colonnades.

aula thermale   Generic term applied to a large hall forming part of a bath complex.

basilica   A structure, often long and rectangular, whose plan consists of a tall central hall, or nave, flanked by side aisles lit by a clerestory, and usually terminating in one or more apses at one end. In Roman times, the basilica was used for various official, and judicial, purposes. The term eventually came to be widely used for any large hall of this plan, regardless of its function.

bema   Chancel section of a Greek or Byzantine church.

Bessi   People of Thrace.

bouleuterion   Small theatre-like structure used for the meetings of a city council (*boule*).

calidarium(-a) or caldarium   The hot room(s) of a Roman bath.

cavea   The seating area of a theatre, or its auditorium, generally divided into a lower (*ima cavea*) and an upper (*summa cavea*) section.

cella   The enclosed central shrine, or chamber, of a Greek or Roman temple, where the statue of the divinity usually stood.

Centaurs   Mythological, wild, part-horse (lower part), part-human (upper body) creatures. Usually considered to be symbols of barbarism. Their fight against the Lapiths (people of Thessaly, in northern Greece, like the Centaurs) are frequent motifs of classical art, hence the term 'Centauromachy' (lit. 'Centaur fight') used in such a context.

chlamydatus   Adjective used for describing the late Roman and early Byzantine male statues of high officials wearing the long (usually woollen) cloak fastened on the right shoulder and fashionable in the fourth and fifth centuries. From *chlamys*, a similar, but shorter cape worn by men in earlier periods.

ciborium   Canopy-like structure placed over a sacred area (altar, throne or tomb) = *baldacchino*.

conch   A semicircular niche, generally featuring a half dome. Hence, *triconch*, a cluster of three conches, or a room featuring a trefoil plan.

conistra   In Roman times, the often deepened area between the stage and the *cavea*, roughly equivalent to the orchestra of classical Greek theatres, but now used as an arena.

contabulatio   Flat group of folds stretched diagonally across the chest in the draping of a toga.

crepis   Stepped platform of a Greek temple. (syn. *crepidoma*.)

cubiculum   Bedroom in a Roman house.

cuneus(-i)   Wedge-shaped unit of the *cavea* of a theatre, divided by radiating passages or flights of steps.

Dacians   People of the lower Danube basin. Their heartland is present-day Rumania.

depas   Drinking cup, goblet or beaker, generally of an elongated shape and flaring body with two large handles. Characteristic 'horizon marker' of Bronze Age Anatolia.

diakonikon   In early Christian context, a room connected to a church, usually serving as vestry or archive.

diazoma(-ata)   Horizontal passageway separating the groups of seats, or upper and lower *caveae*, of a theatre or similar structure.

disjecta membra   (Lat.) lit. 'scattered limbs'. Term used in reference to dispersed material or fragments (statuary, architecture, etc...)

emblema(-ata)   Separately framed panel or section of a mosaic floor or wall.

ependytes   Outer tunic or garment worn over another dress.

extra muros   (Lat.) lit. 'outside the walls'. Outside, beyond walls.

frigidarium   Cold room of a Roman bath.

Giants   Mythological creatures, sons of Gē (Earth) and Uranus. In Hellenistic art, Giants are represented as snake-legged monsters, who challenged and attempted to overthrow the Olympian Gods. A frequent motif in later art, hence the term 'Gigantomachy' (lit. 'Giants fight'), referring to scenes of battle between Gods and Giants.

gymnasium   Exercising ground for athletes and athletic training. Originally part of a school.

Hellenistic   Adjective referring to the period following the death of Alexander the Great (323 BC) up to Octavian's (later Augustus') control of the whole Mediterranean basin (31 BC, Battle of Actium).

heroon   Small shrine, or sanctuary, for a hero, a deified or semi-deified person.

höyük or hüyük   Turkish word referring to an artificial mound created over centuries by successive human habitation, usually consisting of mud brick, or unbaked (sun-dried) brick. Arabic equivalent = *tell*.

hypocaust   A floor system supported by (terracotta) columns in a bath, providing space for the circulation of hot air. A feature of the *calidarium*.

iconostasis   Screen wall decorated with images, or icons, and separating the nave from the chancel (or *bema*) in a Byzantine church.

imago clipeata   (Lat.) lit. 'image, or likeness, in a round frame or disk'. In painting or sculpture, the term is used for a portrait, or other bust, jutting out of a circular frame and used for decoration on walls and pilasters or in niches. Synonymous with *tondo* (round) bust (It.).

in situ   (Lat.) In place; at its original location.

logeion   Platform, or podium (lit. Greek 'speaking place') in a Hellenistic-type theatre stage.

mappa   Handkerchief, or serviette, used for waving (or throwing) by presiding official, as a signal for the start of games and festivities.

monophysite   In the fifth and sixth centuries, adherent to the Christian theological belief that the divine and human elements in Christ are inseparable, with the divine element being dominant. Originated in Alexandria.

naiskos(-i)   Small columnar shrine or niche, projecting in a sequence or a façade arrangement. Diminutive of (Gr.) *naos*, and equivalent of (Lat.) *aedicula*.

naos   (Gr.) Shrine or temple. The word is also used as an equivalent of *cella*.

narthex   An architectural term referring to a transverse vestibule of a church usually preceding the nave and aisles.

Nike   (Gr. 'Victory') Winged goddess symbolizing victory.

nymphaeum   Originally a place dedicated to the nymphs, often a grotto or cave. Eventually, the word applied to all artificial water-filled caves, and especially, a monumental fountain-house with running water.

octastyle   Featuring eight columns on the façade.

odeon   A small theatre building, usually roofed, in which more intimate performances, plays, musical shows and lectures were held. It also was frequently used for official, council meetings. (= *bouleuterion*.)

oecus   (Gr. *oikos*) The main room in a Greek house. In a Roman house, a banqueting room. The word is also often used to refer to an important room in other buildings.

opisthodomos   Back porch of a temple.

opus sectile   Pavement, sometimes wall decoration, consisting of varied, mostly geometric-shaped stone or marble tiles of different colours forming distinctive patterns or figures.

palaestra   Originally, a wrestling school; then, a training school or area intended for athletic exercises. A palaestra was a usual feature of a Roman bath.

parodos(-i)   Side entrance to the orchestra, or *pulpitum*, of a Greek or Roman theatre.

peristyle   Colonnade, or ring of columns surrounding a building.

pithos(-i)   Large (usually terracotta) jars used for the storage of liquids (e.g. watèr, oil or wine) and also drier goods.

porta regia   (Lat.) lit. 'royal door'. The central door of the stage in a Roman theatre.

proedria   Seats of honour, usually in the front row, in a theatre or similar type of structure.

pronaos   The porch in front of the *cella* in a Greek temple.

proskenion   The front portion of the stage of a theatre. Originally, the building in front of the *skene*.

prothesis   A room connected to a church in early Christian times intended for the preparation of the Eucharist before Mass, and its storage afterwards.

pulpitum   Stage portion of a Roman theatre.

scaenae frons   Richly decorated façade of the stage building of a Roman theatre.

Sebasteion   From *Sebastos*, Greek equivalent of Latin Augustus. A place or shrine complex dedicated to the cult of the deified Augustus, and/or other emperors.

Society of Dilettanti   Group of English gentlemen organized in 1734 for the encouragement (at home) of interest in antiquities. The Society sent several expeditions to explore and record antiquities to Greece and Asia Minor between 1764 and 1766. In 1811, under the auspices of the Society, Sir William Gell launched another such expedition. Gell and John Peter Gandy (later Deering), as a draughtsman, visited Aphrodisias between November 1-12, 1812, copying inscriptions, sketching, and measuring the ruins of the ancient city. The results of this work were published in 1840, in the *Antiquities of Ionia*.

stadium   A long (six hundred Greek feet) race course and area framed by seats used for athletic games and contests. The stadium was generally curved at one end. It is curved at both ends at Aphrodisias.

stoa(-i)   A covered portico with a wall at its back and a colonnade in front.

stylobate   Upper step or platform on which the columns of a temple (or other building) rest.

sudatorium   A sweating room in a Roman bath.

synthronon   An arrangement of semicircular rows of seats or benches, often arranged in the apse, or occasionally as straight rows on either side of the chancel, in a Byzantine church. This area was exclusively reserved for church officials.

taberna(-ae) Room or chamber off a building or street, used as a shop.

temenos Sacred precinct or enclosure within which a temple, or group of shrines, were located.

tepidarium 'Lukewarm' hall, or room, in a Roman bath.

tetrapylon Monumental gateway featuring four rows of four columns, or with four equal faces. Often found at the intersection of two streets.

tetrastoon A public area with a *stoa*, or covered portico, on its four sides.

triclinium Originally, the dining-room of a Roman house. (Etymologically, an arrangement of banqueting couches (*klinai*) on three sides of the room.) Eventually, the word came to apply to a reception or principal room, or hall.

via venatorum System of corridors, often parallel to the width of the *pulpitum* and with access doors to the orchestra - *conistra*. This was used as a service or refuge area for hunters, or gladiators, in *venationes* (animal-baiting games) in Roman theatres (or Hellenistic theatres converted for arena or circus-type shows).

vomitorium(-a) Access, as well as exit, corridors of theatres or similar structures.

Architectural Drawings

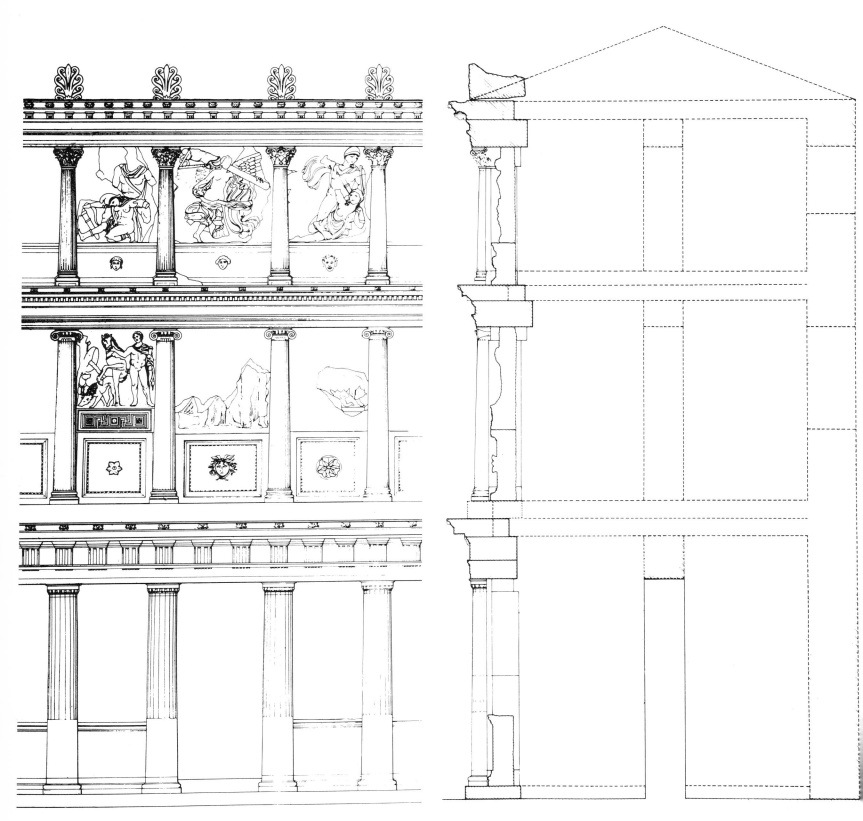

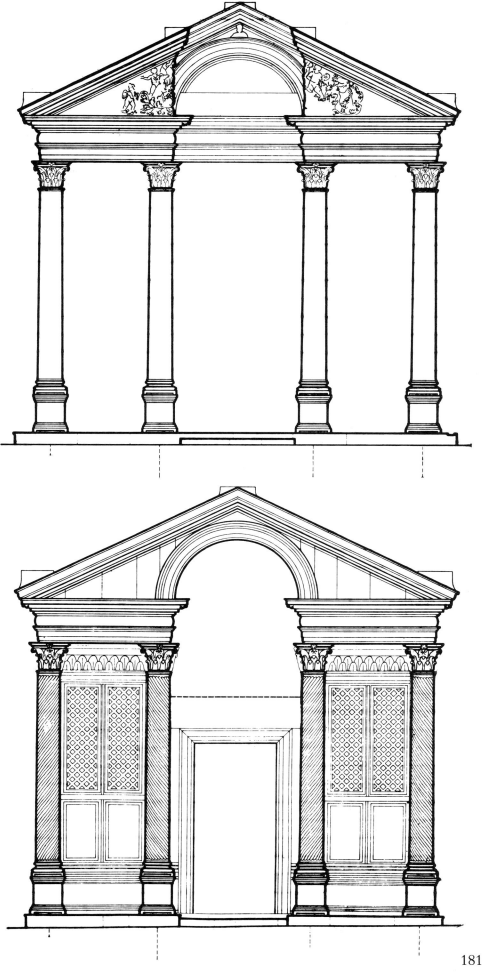

Opposite page
Drawings of the scheme of elevation of the Sebasteion's South Portico show the arrangement of the three superimposed rows of columns. Decorative elements and relief sculptures that have been identified are shown in position to illustrate how the South Portico might have appeared when viewed from the processional way running between the parallel North and South Porticoes.

Left
The Tetrapylon's elegant spirally fluted columns are shown clearly in the lower drawing, which represents the east elevation of the structure. The west elevation is shown in the upper drawing.

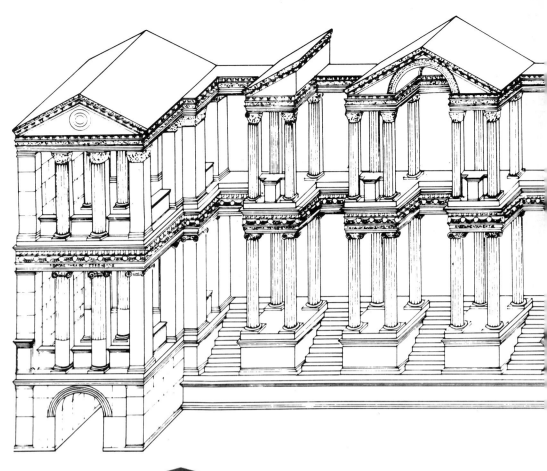

Right
A provisional reconstruction of the so-called 'Agora Gate' illustrates the structure's possible design and gives an indication of its impressive scale and remarkable architectural complexity.

Below
A three-dimensional architectural sketch of the Odeon gives a vivid impression of the elegance of the original structure. The lowest levels remain visible today and still convey a tangible sense of the building's grace and intimacy.

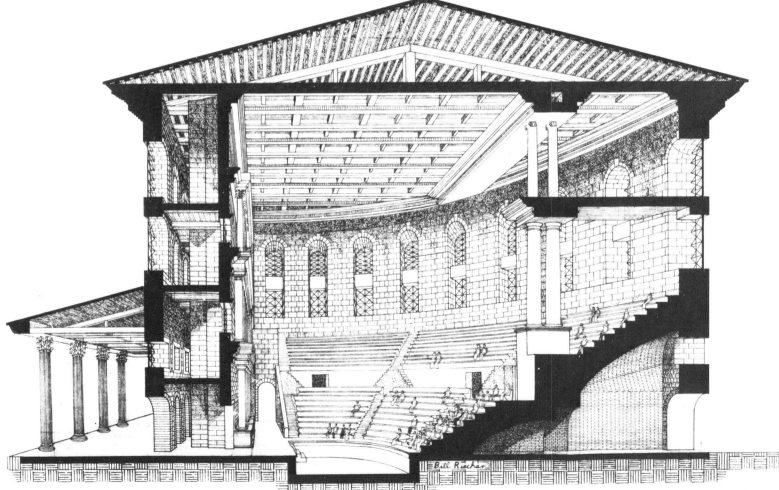

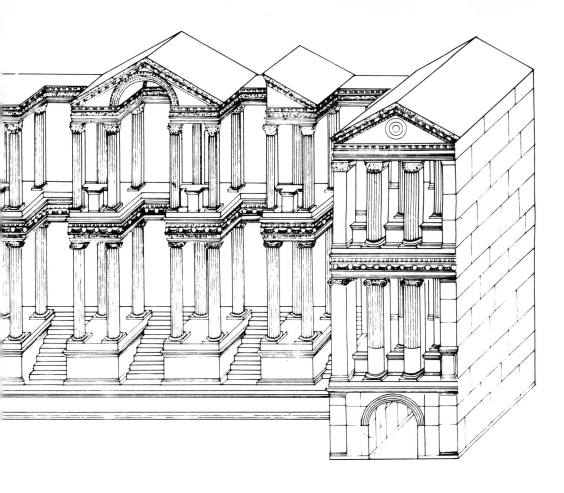

Architectural drawings play an important part in the excavation of
any ancient site. They are valuable as records of exploration and as
measures of progress. They also serve a vital function in providing a
plan — or visual hypothesis — which can be tested against
subsequent discoveries. For this reason several working drawings of
structures excavated at Aphrodisias are shown here, to complete the
picture of the work that is being undertaken. They must be
understood to be provisional, however, as indications of the
thinking at one stage of the project, and are not intended to be
definitive representations. Nevertheless, they offer a view of
structures that cannot be obtained in reality without complete
architectural reconstruction, and so may serve to aid appreciation of
this remarkable and beautiful site.

Bibliographies

BIBLIOGRAPHY LIST OF ABBREVIATIONS

AJA	American Journal of Archaeology.
AJPh	American Journal of Philology.
AnatSt	Anatolian Studies. Journal of the British Institute of Archaeology at Ankara.
Annuario	Annuario della Scuola Archeologica di Atene e delle Missioni Italiane in Oriente.
AntCl	L'antiquité classique.
ArchCl	Archaeologica Classica.
ArchEph	Archaiologike Ephemeris.
BCH	Bulletin de correspondance hellénique. Ecole Française d'Athènes.
Belleten	Belleten. Türk Tarih Kurumu. Ankara.
BdA	Bolletino d'Arte.
BSA	British School at Athens. Annual.
CIG	Corpus Inscriptionum Graecarum.
CR	Classical Review.
CRAI	Comptes Rendus de L'Académie des Inscriptions et Belles-Lettres.
DOPapers	Dumbarton Oaks Papers.
FA	Fasti Archaeologici.
GRBS	Greek, Roman and Byzantine Studies.
HSCP	Harvard Studies in Classical Philology.
ILN	Illustrated London News.
JFA	Journal of Field Archaeology.
JHS	Journal of Hellenic Studies.
JRS	Journal of Roman Studies.
JOAIBeibl	Jahreshefte des Oesterreichischen Archäologischen Instituts. Beiblatt.
LIMC	Lexicon Iconographicum Mythologiae Classicae.
MonAnt	Monumenti Antichi pubblicati per cura della Reale Accademia dei Lincei. Roma.
National Geographic	National Geographic Magazine. Washington, DC.
NC	Numismatic Chronicle.
PBSR or BSR	Papers of the British School at Rome.
ProcBritAc	Proceedings of the British Academy.
RA	Revue archéologique.
RE	A. Pauly and B. Wissowa. Real-encyclopädie der classischen Altertumwissenschaft, Stuttgart.

REA	Revue des études anciennes.
REG	Revue des études grecques.
RendPontAcc	Rendiconti della Pontifica Accademia Romana di Archaeologica.
RevPhil	Revue de Philologie. Nouvelle Série.
RömMitt	Mitteilungen des Deutschen Archäologischen Instituts. Römische Abteilung.
TürkArkDerg	Türk Arkeoloji Dergisi.
ZPE	Zeitschrift für Papyrologie und Epigraphik.
ZRG	Zeitschrift der Savigny-Stiftung für Rechtsgeschichte (or Zeitschrift für Rechtsgeschichte).

SELECT APHRODISIAS BIBLIOGRAPHY
PRIOR TO CURRENT EXCAVATIONS

1   Early Travel Accounts and reports.

Antiquities of Ionia, Society of Dilettanti, London, III, 1840, pls. I-XXIV.

Ch. Fellows, *An Account of Discoveries in Lycia*, London, 1841, p.32.

W.J. Hamilton, *Researches in Asia Minor, Pontus and Armenia* London, 1842, p.529.

Ch. Texier, *Description de l'Asie Mineure*, Paris, III, 1849, pp. 149ff, pls. 150ff.

L. de Laborde, *Voyage de l'Asie Mineure*, Paris, 1872, pl. 53

G. Hirschfeld, in *Monatsberichte der preussische Akademie in Berlin*, 1879, p. 328.

A. Kubitschek and W. Reichel, "Reise in Karien", *Anzeiger Wiener Akademie*, XXX (1893), pp. 92-105.

2   General Accounts

G. Hirschfeld, in Pauly-Wissowa *RE*, 1894, I^2, 2726.

R. Vagts, *Aphrodisias in Karien*, Diss., Hamburg, 1920.

G. Becatti, in *Enciclopedia dell'Arte Antica, Classica e Orientale*, Rome, 1958, I, pp. 109-115

3   Early Excavations.

M. Collignon, in *CRAI*, (1904), pp. 703-11; in *Revue de l'Art Ancien et Moderne*, XIX (1906), pp. 33ff.

G. Mendel, in *CRAI* (1906), pp. 178-84.

A. Boulanger, in *CRAI* (1914), pp. 46ff.

Th. Reinach, *REG* XIX (1906), pp. 79-150 and 205-98. [Inscriptions].

G. Mendel, *Catalogue des sculptures grecques, romaines et byzantines, Musées Impériaux Ottomans de Constantinople*, Constantinople, III, 1914, pp. 176-213.

G. Jacopi, in *ILN*, 18 December 1937, pp. 1095-97.

G. Jacopi "Gli scavi della Missione Archaeologica Italiana ad Afrodisiade" and L. Crema, "I monumenti architettonia afrodisiensi", in MonAnt, 38 (1939-40).

E. Will, in *RA*, 12 (1938), pp. 228ff.

4   *Sculpture and Related Publications.*

E. Löwy, *Inschriften griechischer Bildhauer*, Leipzig, 1885, pp. 25-9; pp. 268-9 and p. 375.

G. Lippold, *Kopien und Umbildungen griechischer Statuen*, Munich, 1923, *passim*.

J. M. C. Toynbee, *The Hadrianic School*, Cambridge, 1934, *passim*.

M. Squarciapino, *La Scuola di Afrodisia*, Rome, 1943.

J. M. C. Toynbee and J. B. Ward-Perkins, in *BSR*, 18 (1950) pp. 1ff.

J. M. C. Toynbee, *Some Notes on Artists in the Roman World*, Collection Latomus, Brussels, VI, (1951), pp. 29ff.

J. B. Ward-Perkins, in *ProcBritAc*, 38 (1951), pp. 269ff.

G. M. A. Richter, *Three Critical Periods in Greek Sculpture*, Oxford, 1951, *passim*.

E. Will, *Le relief cultuel gréco-romain*, Paris, 1955, pp. 448ff.

A. Dönmez, in *ILN*, 25 April 1959, pp. 712-13.

A. Giuliano, in *Annuario*, 37-8 (1959-60), pp. 389ff.

5   *Cult and Cult-Statue of Aphrodite*

C. Friedrich, in *RömMitt*, XXII (1897), pp. 361ff.

F. Magi, in *RendPontAcc*, XII (1936), pp. 221ff.

H. Thiersch, *Ependytes und Ephod*, Stuttgart, 1937.

R. Schilling, *La religion romaine de Vénus*, Paris, 1954, *passim*.

F. Eichler, *JOAIBeibl*, 42 (1955), pp. 1-22.

A. Laumonier, *Les cultes indigènes en Carie*, Paris, 1958, pp. 478ff.

M. Squarciapino, in *BdA*, XLIV (1959), pp. 97ff.; *ArchCl*, XII, 2 (1960) pp. 208ff; *RendPontAcc*, XXXVIII (1965-6), pp. 143ff.

6   Miscellaneous. History, Topography

D. Magie, *Roman Rule in Asia Minor*, Princeton, 1950, *passim*.

E. Honigmann, *Evêques et évêchés monophysites d'Asie antérieure au VIème siècle*, Louvain, 1951, *passim*.

L. and J. Robert, *La Carie. Histoire et géographie historique. Tome II. Le plateau de Tabae et ses environs*, Paris, 1954, *passim*.

7   Inscriptions, Epigraphical and Related Studies.

Most of the early travel accounts include transcriptions of inscriptions. For the epigraphical material collected by the 1904-5 excavations, see under *3. Early Excavations*, Th. Reinach's articles in *REG*.

W. Leake (from Gandy/Deering's copies of 1812), in *Transactions of the Royal Society of Literature in the United Kingdom*, 1843, pp. 232ff.

CIG, 1843, nos. 2737-2851, with pp. 1109-19, and nos. 8633, 8643, 8919 and 9729.

P. Le Bas and W. H. Waddington, *Inscriptions grecques et latines recueillies en Grèce et en Asie Mineure*, 1870, nos. 589-96 and 1585-1650.

J. R. S. Sterrett, *An Epigraphical Journey in Asia Minor* (Papers of the American School of Classical Studies at Athens, II, 1883-4) 1888, nos. 9, 10.

P. Paris and M. Holleaux, in *BCH*, 9 (1885), pp. 68ff.; G. Radet, in BCH, 14 (1890), pp. 224ff.; G. Doublet and G. Deschamps, also in *BCH*, 14 (1890), pp. 610ff.

H. Grégoire, *Recueil des inscriptions grecques chrétiennes d'Asie Mineure*, 1922, nos. 246-281 bis.

A. Salač, in *BCH*, 51 (1927) pp. 236ff.

L. Robert, in *BCH*, 52 (1928), p. 414; in *RA*, 30, 1929, p,28; in *RevPhil*, 55 (1929), p. 126; in *RevPhil*, 56 (1930), pp. 25ff.

W. M. Calder, in CR, 49 (1935), pp. 216ff.

L. Robert, in *Etudes Anatoliennes*, 1937, *passim*; and in *Anatolian Studies Presented to W. H. Buckler*, 1939, pp. 230ff.

Relevant items and observations on Aphrodisias and its inscriptions can usually be found in J. and L. Robert, "Bulletin Epigraphique", published in *REG*, from 1938 on.

L. Robert, *Les gladiateurs dans l'orient grec*, Paris, 1940, *passim*.

L. Robert, in *Hellenica*, IV (1948), pp. 47ff.; pp. 115ff. and 127ff.; XI-XII (1960) pp. 46ff.; in *REA*, 62 (1960), p. 291.

J. M. R. Cormack, *Notes on the History of the Inscribed Monuments of Aphrodisias*, Reading, 1955.

W. M. Calder and J. M. R. Cormack, in *Monumenta Asiae Minoris Antigua, VIII: Monuments from Lycaonia the Pisido-Phrygian Border, Aphrodisias,* Manchester, 1962, pp. 72-160.

L. Robert, *Villes d'Asie Mineure,* Paris, 1962, pp. 64, 66, 82, 106, 217, 326, 421.

L. Robert, *Noms indigènes dans l'Asie Mineure gréco-romaine,* 1ᵉʳ partie, Paris, 1963.

J. M. R. Cormack, in *BSA,* 59 (1964), pp. 16ff.

E. Lane, in *Berytus,* 15 (1964), pp. 27-8.

L. Robert, in *Hellenica,* 13 (1965), pp. 109ff.; in *Gnomon,* 37, 1965, pp. 381ff.; in *AntCl,* 35.(1966), pp. 377; in *ArchEph,* 1966, pp. 113-5.

P. Veyne, in *Mélanges Piganiol,* 1966, pp. 1395-6.

J. Ebert, in *Zeitschrift Marthin Luther Universität Halle/Wittenberg,* 15 (1966), pp. 375ff.

RECENT APHRODISIAS BIBLIOGRAPHY

K. T. Erim, "Classical and Christian Discoveries in the Carian City of Aphrodisias — At the Beginning of new Excavations" (Archaeological Section No. 2076), *ILN,* January 13, 1962, pp. 61-63.

K. T. Erim, "Further Findings from the Carian 'Mine of Statuary': and the Discovery of the Unique Cult Statue of Aphrodisias", (Archaeological Section No. 2118), *ILN,* January 5, 1963, pp. 20-23.

K. T. Erim, "More Treasures from the 'Mine of Statuary': Excavations at Aphrodisias in Caria in Southwest Turkey. Part I: The Temple and the Odeon", (Archaeological Section No. 2163), *ILN,* December 21, 1963, pp. 1028-31.

K. T. Erim, "Excavations in the Roman and Byzantine City. Part II: Buildings and Still More Statuary", (Archaeological Section No. 2164), *ILN,* December 28, 1963, pp. 1066-1069.

K. T. Erim, "The 'Mine of Statuary' in Aphrodisias", (Archaeological Section No. 2213), *ILN,* February 20, 1965, pp. 21-23.

K. T. Erim, "Odeon and Statuary at Aphrodisias", (Archaeological Section No. 2214), *ILN,* February 27, 1965, pp. 22-23.

K. T. Erim, "Aphrodisias Excavations, 1964", *Archaeology,* 18, 1, 1965, pp. 67-68.

K. T. Erim "Atelier to the Empire", *Horizon,* March 1960, pp. 96-100.

K. T. Erim, in *TürkArkDerg,* 11-2 (1961), pp. 26-29; 12-1 (1962), pp. 14-18; 13-2 (1964), pp. 86-92; 14-2 (1965), pp. 135-140; 15-1 (1966), pp. 59-67; 15-2 (1966), pp. 55-59; 16-1 (1967), pp. 67-80; 17-1 (1968), pp. 43-57; 18-2 (1970), pp. 87-93; 20-1 (1973), pp. 63-87; 21-1 (1974), pp. 37-57; 22-2 (1975), pp. 73-92; 23-1 (1976), pp. 25-50; 25-1 (1980), pp. 15-38.

K. T. Erim, in M. J. Mellink, "Archaeology in Asia Minor", *AJA,* 67 (1963), pp. 184-85; 68 (1964), pp. 160-61; 69 (1965), p. 145; 70 (1966), pp. 154-55; 71

(1967), pp. 155 and 171-72; 72 (1968), pp. 131-32 and 142-44; 73 (1969), pp. 208-09 and 223-24; 74 (1970), pp. 163 and 174; 75 (1971), pp. 177-78; 76 (1972), pp. 172 and 184-85; 77 (1973), pp. 174 and 188-89; 78 (1974), pp. 126-27; 79 (1975), pp. 219-20; 80 (1976), pp. 277-78; 81 (1977), pp. 296 and 305-06; 82 (1978), pp. 317 and 324-25; 83 (1979), pp. 338-39; 84 (1980), pp. 505, 511; 85 (1981), pp. 471-72; 86 (1982), pp. 568-69; 87 (1983), pp. 438-39; 88 (1984), p. 454.

K. T. Erim, in D. H. French, *et al.* "Recent Archaeological Research in Turkey", *AnatSt*, XIV (1964), pp. 25-28, XVI (1966), pp. 36-39; XVIII (1968), pp. 32-36; XIX (1969), pp. 14-16; XX (1970), pp. 20-24; XXI (1971), pp. 25-31; XXII (1972), pp. 35-40; XXIII (1973), pp. 19-24; XXIV (1974), pp. 20-23; XXV (1975), pp. 17-22; XXVI (1976), pp. 24-30; XXVII (1977), pp. 29-32; XXVIII (1978), pp. 10-13 XXIX (1979), pp. 186-88; XXX (1980), pp. 205-06; XXXI (1981), pp. 177-81; XXXII (1982), pp. 9-13; XXXIII, pp. 231-35.

K. T. Erim, in H. Alkim, "Exploration and Excavation in Turkey 1963", *Jaarbericht. Ex Oriente Lux*, 18 (1964), pp. 371-72: *Anatolica* I (1967), pp. 29-30; II (1968), pp. 52-55; III (1970), pp. 48-53; IV (1971-1972), pp. 40-44.

K. T. Erim, in *FA*, XVI (1961), 3698, p. 261; XVII (1962), 3810-11, pp. 267-68; XVIII-XIX (1963-1964), 5822, pp. 416-19; XX (1965), 3622, pp. 240-43; XXI (1966) 2870, p. 202 and 3387, p. 236; XXII (1967) 3382-83, p. 267; XXIII (1968), 3389-90, pp. 244-50; XXIV-XXV (1969-1970), 6466-67, pp. 442-45; XXVIII-XXIX (1973-1974), 7845-47, pp. 495-503; XXX-XXXI (1975-1976), 9320-21, pp. 632-37.

J. Inan and Elisabeth Rosenbaum, *Roman and Early Byzantine Portrait Sculpture in Asia Minor*, London, 1966, pp. 4, 6, 11, 18, 30-34 (*passim*); 36, 40ff., 43, 84, 89-90, 171-75, 177-82.

K. T. Erim, "De Aphrodisiade", *AJA*, 71 (1967), pp. 233-43.

K. T. Erim "The School of Aphrodisias", *Archaeology*, 20, 1, January 1967, pp. 18-27.

K. T. Erim, "Two New Early Byzantine Statues from Aphrodisias" and I. Ševčenko, "An Epigram Honoring the *Praeses* of Caria, Oikoumenios", *DOPapers* 21 (1967), pp. 285-86.

K. T. Erim, "Aphrodisias and Its Marble Treasures", *National Geographic*, 132, August 1967, pp. 280-94.

K. T. Erim, "Roman and Early Byzantine Portrait Sculpture in Asia Minor Supplement I", *Belleten*, 32, 125 (1968), pp. 4-18. (With J. Inan and E. Alföldi).

I. Ševčenko, "A Late Epigram and the so-called Elder Magistrate from Aphrodisias", *Synthronon*. Art et archéologie de la fin de l'Antiquité et du Moyen âge. Recueil d'études par Andrè Grabar et un groupe de ses disciples, Paris, 1968, pp. 29-41.

K. T. Erim and J. M. Reynolds, "A Letter of Gordian III from Aphrodisias in Caria", *JRS*, 59 (1969), pp. 56-58.

K. T. Erim, "Aphrodisias" in E. Akurgal, *Ancient Civilisations and Ruins of Turkey*, Istanbul, 1969, pp. 171-75.

D. J. de Solla Price, "Portable Sundials in Antiquity, including an Account of a New Example from Aphrodisias", *Centaurus* 14 (1969), pp. 242-66.

K. T. Erim, "Two New Inscriptions from Aphrodisias", *PBSR*, 37 (1969), pp. 92-95.

S. Pancera, "Miscellanea epigraphica", *Epigrafica*, 31 (1969) pp. 112-20.

L. Robert, in J. des Gagniers (ed.), *Laodicée du Lycos*, Paris, 1969, p. 302.

B. Kadish (with K. T. Erim), "Excavations of Prehistoric Remains at Aphrodisias, 1967", *AJA*, 73 (1969), pp. 49-65.

K. T. Erim and J. M. Reynolds, "The Copy of Diocletian's Edict on Maximum Prices from Aphrodisias in Caria", *JRS*, 60 (1970), pp. 120-41.

189

K. T. Erim, "Three Portraits from Aphrodisias", *Studies in Honor of J. Alexander Kerns*, The Hague, 1970, pp. 25-28.

O. Carruba, "A Lydian Inscription from Aphrodisias in Caria", *JHS*, 90 (1970), pp. 195-96.

W. Seston, "La citoyenneté romaine", *XIIème Congrès des Sciences Humaines*, II (1970), pp. 48-49.

J. H. Oliver, "A Rescript of Gordian III to L. Aurelius Epaphras", *GRBS*, 11 (1970), pp. 137-38.

G. Bowersock, in a review of R. K. Sherk, *Roman Documents from the Greek East, AJPh*, 91 (1970), pp. 225-26.

L. Robert, in a review of F. G. Maier, *Mauerinschriften, Gnomon*, 42 (1970), pp. 591-92.

R. Merkelbach, "Herakles und der Pankratiast", *ZPE*, 6 (1970), pp. 47-49; and "Epigramm aus Aphrodisias", *ZPE*, 6 (1970), p. 132.

B. Kadish (with K. T. Erim), "Excavations of Prehistoric Remains at Aphrodisias, 1968 and 1969", *AJA*, 75 (1971), pp. 121-40.

K. T. Erim, J. M. Reynolds and M. Crawford, "Diocletian's Currency Reform. A New Inscription from Aphrodisias", *JRS*, 61 (1971) pp. 171-77.

T. Drew-Bear, "Deux inscriptions à Aphrodisias", *ZPE*, 8 (1971), pp. 285-88.

L. Robert, "Les colombes d'Anastase et autres volatiles", *Journal des Savants*, 1971, pp. 91-97.

T. Ritti, "Gare di scultura ad Afrodisia", *RendAccLinc*, 1971, pp. 189-94.

M. Wörrle, "Ägyptisches Getreide für Ephesos", *Chiron*, 1 (1971), p. 332.

Speros Vryonis, Jr., *The Decline of Medieval Hellenism in Asia Minor and the Process of Islamization from the eleventh through the fifteenth century*, Berkeley, 1971, *passim*.

K. T. Erim, "The Ninth Campaign of Excavations at Aphrodisias in Caria, 1969", VII. *Türk Tarih Kurumu Kongresi Bildirileri, Ankara 1970, Vol. I*, Ankara, 1972, pp. 155-60.

T. Drew-Bear, "Deux décrets hellénistiques d'Asie Mineure", *BCH*, 96 (1972), pp. 435-71.

J. H. Oliver, "On the Hellenic Policy of Augustus and Agrippa,"in 27 BC *AJPh*, 93 (1972), pp. 195-97.

K. T. Erim and J. M. Reynolds, "The Aphrodisias Copy of Diocletian's Edict on Maximum Prices", *JRS*, 63 (1973), pp. 99-110.

J. M. Reynolds, "Aphrodisias, a Free and Federate City", *Vestigia*, 17 (1973), pp. 115-22.

F. G. Millar, "Triumvirate and Principate", *JRS*, 63 (1973), p. 50-58.

K. T. Erim, "The 'Acropolis' of Aphrodisias in Caria: Investigations of the Theater and the Prehistoric Mounds 1966-1967", *National Geographic Society Research Reports*, Washington, DC., 1973, pp. 89-112.

K. T. Erim, "A Portrait Statue of Domitian from Aphrodisias", *Opuscula Romana*, IX (1973), pp. 135-42.

K. T. Erim "Afrodisiade" article in *Supplemento: Enciclopedia dell'Arte Antica, classica e Orientale*, Rome, 1973, pp. 9-17.

K. T. Erim, "The Satyr and Young Dionysus Group from Aphrodisias," *Mélanges Mansel*, Ankara, 1974, pp. 767-75.

K. T. Erim "Afrodisias", in D. de Bernardi Ferrero, *Teatri classici in Asia Minore*, Vol. IV, Rome, 1974, pp. 162-66.

D. J. MacDonald, "Aphrodisias and Currency in the East, AD 259-305", *AJA*, 78 (1974), pp. 279-86.

K. T. Erim and D. J. MacDonald, "A Hoard of Alexander Drachms", *NC*, IV (1974), pp. 171-73.

H. J. Wieling, "Eine neuentdeckte Inschrift Gordians III und ihre Bedeutung für das Verständnis der *Constitutio Antoniniana*", *ZRG*, 91 (1974), pp. 364-74.

R. Merkelbach, "Ueber ein ephesisches Dekret für einen Athleten aus Aphrodisias", *ZPE*, 14 (1974), pp. 91-96.

R. Merkelbach, "Nochmal zum Dekret für den Pankratiasten Kallikrates", *ZPE*, 15 (1974), p. 276.

L. Robert, "Des Carpathes à la Propontide", *Studii Clasice*, 16 (1974), p. 76.

E. Berger, "La reconstruction du groupe d'Achille et Penthésilée", *RA* (Bulletin de la S.F.A.C.) I (1976), pp.187-189.

D. J. MacDonald, *Greek and Roman Coins from Aphrodisias* (British Archaeological Reports, Series 9), Oxford, 1976.

K. T. Erim, "Aphrodisias", *Princeton Encyclopedia of Classical Sites*, Princeton, 1976, pp. 68-70.

K. T. Erim, "The 'Acropolis' of Aphrodisias in Caria: Investigations of the Theater and the Prehistoric Mounds, 1968-1970", *National Geographic Society Research Reports*, 1968 Projects, Washington, DC., 1976, pp. 79-113.

R. T. Marchese, "Report on West Acropolis Excavations at Aphrodisias, 1971-1973", *AJA*, 80 (1976), pp. 393-413.

A. Cameron, *Circus Factions: Blues and Greens at Rome and Byzantium*, Oxford, 1976, pp. 314-19.

K. T. Erim, "Aphrodisias", *Istanbul Hilton Magazine*, Fall 1977, pp. 14-19.

F. G. Millar, *The Emperor in the Roman World, (31 BC-AD 337)*. Ithaca, 1977, pp. xiii, 243, 343, 414, 416, 417, 429, 431-32, 438-39, 480 and 614.

V. Nutton, "Archiatri and the Medical Profession", *PBSR*, 45 (1977), nos. 1-3, pp. 192ff.

L. Robert, "Documents d'Asie Mineure", *BCH*, 101 (1977), pp. 86-88.

M. I. Finley (ed.), *Atlas of Classical Archaeology*, New York, 1977, pp. 210-11.

K. T. Erim "Recent Discoveries at Aphrodisias", and "Sculpture from Aphrodisias", pp. 1063-84.

J. M. Reynolds, "The Inscriptions of Aphrodisias", pp. 627-34, *Proceedings of the Tenth International Congress of Classical Archaeology Vol. II*, Ankara, 1978.

M. S. Joukowsky, "Computer Use in Pottery Studies at Aphrodisias", *JFA*, 5 (1978), pp. 431-42.

M. F. Squarciapino, "Rintrovamenti archeologici all'estro: Gli scavi di Aphrodisias di Caria", *Studi Romani*, 26.3 (1978), pp. 348-89.

K. T. Erim, in J. Inan and E. Alföldi-Rosenbaum, *Römische und frühbyzantinische Porträtplastik aus der Türkei. Neue Funde*, Mainz a. R. 1979, pp. 6-7; 78-79; 82-83; 89-91; 100-01; 111-12; 126-27; 134-35; 202-238 and 301-02.

K. T. Erim "The Zoilos Frieze", J. M. Reynolds, "Zoilos: The Epigraphic Evidence", in A. Alföldi, *Aion in Mérida und Aphrodisias* (Madrider Beiträge, 6), Mainz a. R., 1979, pp. 35-40.

K. T. Erim, *Aphrodisias. A Guide Book*. Izmir, 1979.

K. T. Erim, "Aphrodisias. A New Museum", *Istanbul Hilton Magazine*, Winter 1979, pp. 5-7.

K. T. Erim, "Afrodisias ve Heykelcilik", *Yaçar Holding, A. Ş. Bilim, Birlik, Başari*, 1979, pp. 15-22.

S. Mitchell and A. W. McNicoll, "Archaeology in Western and Southern Asia Minor", *Archaeological Reports for 1978-79*, London, 1979, pp. 75-78.

C. M. Roueché, "A New Inscription from Aphrodisias and the Title πατὴρ τῆς πόλεως", *GRBS*, 20, 2, Summer 1979, pp. 173-85.

J. M. Reynolds, "The Aphrodisias copy of Diocletian's Edict on Maximum Prices", *ZPE*, 33 (1979), p. 46.

M. Crawford and J. M. Reynolds, "The Aezani Copy of Diocletian's Edict on Maximum Prices", *ZPE*, 34 (1979), pp. 197, 203 and 206.

A. D. Macro, "A Confirmed Asiarch", *AJPh*, 100 (1979), pp. 94-98.

G. Bean, *Turkey Beyond the Maeander*, London, 1980, pp. 188-98.

K. T. Erim, "The 'Acropolis' of Aphrodisias in Caria. Investigations of the

Theater and Prehistoric Mounds, 1971-1977", *National Geographic Society Research Reports, 1971, Projects*, 12, Washington, DC., 1980, pp. 185-204.

L. Robert, *A travers l'Asie Mineure*, Poètes et prosateurs. Monnaies grecques. Voyageurs et géographie, Paris, 1980

J. M. Reynolds, "The Origins and Beginnings of the Imperial Cult at Aphrodisias", *Proceedings of the Cambridge Philological Society,* 206 (1980), pp. 70-84.

W. Peck, "Griechische Versinchriften aus Kleinasien", *Denkschrift Akad. Wien*, 143 (1980), p. 28.

K. T. Erim, "Aphrodisias 1979", *II. Kazi Sonuçlari Toplantisi*, Ankara, 1980, pp. 37-39.

K. T. Erim, "Ancient Aphrodisias Lives Through its Art," *National Geographic*, 160 (October 1981) pp. 526-51.

C. Roueché, "Rome, Asia and Aphrodisias in the Third Century", *JRS*, 71 (1981), pp. 103-20.

J. M. Reynolds, "Diocletian's Edict on Maximum Prices: The Chapter on Wool", *ZPE*, 42 (1981), p. 283.

J. M. Reynolds, "New Evidence for the Imperial Cult in Julio-Claudian Aphrodisias", *ZPE*, 43 (1981), pp. 317-27.

Evelyn B. Harrison, "Motifs of the City-Siege on the Shield of Athena Parthenos", *AJA*, 85 (1981), pp. 281-317 *passim*.

C. P. Jones, "Two Inscriptions from Aphrodisias", *HSCP*, 85 (1981), pp. 107-29.

K. T. Erim, "Andreia", *LIMC*, I, 1, Zürich and Münich, 1981, p. 764.

P. Pattenden, "A Late Sundial at Aphrodisias", *JHS*, 101 (1981), pp. 101-12.

R. Cormack, "The Classical Tradition in the Byzantine Provincial City. The Evidence of Thessalonike and Aphrodisias", *Byzantium and the Classical Tradition*, Birmingham, 1981, pp. 103-19.

K. T. Erim, "Aphrodisias 1980", *III. Kazi Sonuçlari Toplantisi*, Ankara, 1981, pp. 21-24.

W. Eck, "Miscellanea Prosopographica", *ZPE*, 42 (1981), pp. 235-40.

M. H. Quet, "Aiōn, à propos d'un livre récent", *REA*, 83 (1981), 1-2, pp. 97-108.

J. M. Reynolds, *Aphrodisias and Rome* (*JRS* Monograph I), London, 1982.

K. T. Erim, "A Relief showing Claudius and Britannia from Aphrodisias", *Britannia*, 13 (1982), pp. 277-81.

K. T. Erim, "Récentes découvertes à Aphrodisias en Carie, 1979-1980", *RA* (Bulletin de la SFAC XIV-1980-1981), I (1982), pp. 163-69.

C. Roueché and K. T. Erim, "Sculptors from Aphrodisias: Some New Inscriptions", *PBSR*, 50 (1982), pp. 102-15.

T. Cornell and J. Matthews, *Atlas of the Roman World*, Oxford, 1982, p. 154 and 157.

S. Price, "Aphrodite's City in Turkey", *Omnibus*, 4, November 1982, pp. 1-3.

M. S. Joukowsky, "Late Chalcolithic Figurines from Aphrodisias in Southwestern Turkey", *Archéologie au Levant*, Recueil R. Saidah, 12 (1982), pp. 87-94.

K. T. Erim, "Aphrodisias 1981", *IV. Kazi Sonuçlari Toplantisi*, Ankara, 1982, p. 55.

K. T. Erim, "Aphrodisias", *1981 Excavations in Turkey*, Ankara, 1982, pp. 55.

K. T. Erim, "Aphrodisias", *Hallmark, Archaeology in Turkey Today*, Ankara, 1982, pp. 27-32.

K. T. Erim, "Aphrodisias 1982", *V. Kazi Sonuçlari Toplantisi*, Ankara 1983, pp. 275-83.

L. Robert, "Documents d'Asie Mineure", *BCH*, 107 (1983), pp. 509-11.

K. T. Erim, "The Lure of Aphrodisias", *Pacific Northwest*, 17, 5 (1983), pp. 56-57.

N. de Chaisemartin and E. Örgen, "Les sculptures de Silahtaraga", *RA* (Bulletin de la SFAC), I (1983), pp. 181-89.

F. Işik "Kleinasiatische Girlandsarkophage mit Pilaster-oder Säulenarchitektur", *JOAIBeibl*, 51 (1983), pp. 30-146.

K. M Hendrigks, "Aphrodisias and Rome, Doc. I.", *Epigraphica Anatolica*, III (1984), pp. 33-35.

W. Orth, "Der Triumvir Octavian...", *Epigraphica Anatolica*, III (1984), pp. 61-82.

K. T. Erim, "Aphrodisias", *LIMC*, II, 1, Zürich and Münich, 1984, pp. 1-2.

F. Işik, "Die Sarkophage von Aphrodisias", *Marburger Winckelmann-Programm*, 1984, pp. 243-81.

J. Linderski, "Rome, Aphrodisias and the *Res Gestae*: The *Genera Militiae* and the Status of Octavian", *JRS*, 74 (1984), pp. 74-80.

C. Roueché, "Acclamations in the Later Roman Empire: New Evidence from Aphrodisias", JRS, 74 (1984), pp. 181-99.

S. R. F. Price, *Rituals and Power. The Roman Imperial Cult in Asia Minor*, Cambridge, 1984, pp. 41, 83, 118-19, 127, 137 and 261.

Reviews of J. M. Reynolds, *Aphrodisias and Rome*, London, 1982:

A. N. Sherwin-White, in *JRS*, 73 (1983), pp. 220-22.

G. W. Bowersock, in *Gnomon*, 56 (1984), pp. 48-53.

S. Mitchell, in *CR*, 34 (1984), pp. 291-97.

K. Rigsby, in *Phoenix*, 38 (1984), pp. 102-04.

M. S. Joukowsky (*et al.*) *Prehistoric Aphrodisias. An Account of the Excavations and Artifact Studies.* (Publications d'Histoire de l'Art et d'Archéologie de l'Université Catholique de Louvain. 40. Archaeologica Transatlantica), Providence, R. I., Louvain-la-Neuve, 1983.

Frequent relevant items and brief comments in J. and L. Robert, "Bulletin épigraphique", *REG*:

1961, no. 666; 1963, no. 249; 1965, no. 364; 1966, nos. 380-418; 1967, nos. 539-554; 1968, nos. 507-08; 1969, nos. 541-43; 1970, nos. 530-39; 1971, nos. 609-16; 1972, nos. 413-15; 1973, nos. 398-401; 1974, nos. 532-34; 1976, no. 633; 1977, nos. 459-60; 1978, no. 448; 1979, no. 447; 1981, nos. 516-18; 1982, nos. 355-60; 1983, nos. 361-94.

Index

In this index references to illustrations and their captions are printed in italic.

Picture Credits

The Publishers would like to thank the following for their photographic contributions to this book. Photographs are identified by page number, and by the letters a, b, c etc. denoting the location of photographs on the page, from left to right and top to bottom.

Jonathan S. Blair: ii/iii, 2, 5, 6, 8, 9a, 9b, 10, 19, 20, 21, 31, 36, 39a, 39b, 40b, 41a, 41b, 41c, 43a, 43b, 43c, 46, 49a, 49b, 52, 55b, 60, 61c, 65c, 66b, 68, 75, 77a, 77b, 78a, 78b, 82c, 87, 97c, 122b, 125, 132, 138, 140a, 140b, 140c, 141c, 142a, 142b, 142c, 143, 144b, 146b, 147c, 151a, 154a, 154b, 155a, 157a, 160. **David L. Brill:** i, viii, 11, 14, 24, 53, 54, 55a, 56, 59, 62, 67, 69b, 71, 73, 74, 76, 81, 82, 83b, 85a, 85b, 86b, 89, 92, 94, 97b, 99, 100b, 101c, 101d, 102, 103a, 103b, 103c, 104a, 104b, 105a, 105b, 107a, 113, 114a, 114b, 115a, 115c, 117a, 117c, 124, 126a, 126b, 137a, 137b, 138b, 139a, 139b, 140d, 141a, 141b, 142d, 147a, 147b, 151, 152, 155b, 155c, 156a, 156b, 156c, 156d, 157b, 173. **British Museum/Antiquities of Ionia:** 38a. **M. Ali Döğenci:** vi, 26, 27, 28, 30, 40, 45a, 45b, 58, 61a, 61b, 63a, 64a, 64b, 65a, 65b, 66a, 69a, 82c, 82d, 83a, 84, 86a, 90a, 90b, 91a, 91b, 93, 94b, 96, 97a, 98a, 98b, 101b, 108, 110a, 110b, 111a, 111b, 111c, 112, 115b, 116a, 116b, 117b, 118c, 120a, 120b, 121a, 121c, 122a, 123, 128a, 128b, 129b, 129c, 135, 136, 144a, 144c, 146a, 148a, 148b, 148c, 150, 151b, 158, 159b. **Kenan T. Erim:** 3, 4, 23, 50, 57, 63b, 72, 100, 106a, 106b, 109a, 109b, 118b, 127b, 134, 149, 159. **Paul Gaudin/ courtesy of Albert Gaudin:** 38b, 42, 44a, 44b. **Justin M. Gorence:** 101a, 118a, 119, 121b, 127a, 129a. **Hal Robinson:** 131. **Adam Woolfit:** 63c, 140e, 147b.

The photographs by Jonathan Blair, David Brill and Adam Woolfit are reprinted by courtesy of National Geographic Society.

The photograph of the author on page 200 was taken by Cecil Beaton when he visited Aphrodisias in 1964. It is reproduced from an original print owned privately by Madeleine Chalette Lejwa, in New York. The author and the Publishers would like to acknowledge the assistance of the Cecil Beaton Archive (courtesy of Sotheby's, London) and Vogue/Condé Nast Publications Inc.

The poem *Ruins at Sunset* is printed with kind permission of L. G. Harvey.

The maps on pages 16/17, 32/33, 51 and 107 are by Jeff Edwards, of Marlborough Design, Oxford.

The architectural drawings on pages 180 to 183 are reproduced by courtesy of F. Hueber and U. Outscher (180), F. Hueber and G. Paul (180), B. Rose and D. Theodorescu (182/183) and W. Rischar (182).

Kenan T. Erim

The son of a Turkish diplomat, Kenan T. Erim was educated in Switzerland then enrolled at New York University in 1948, when his father joined the United Nations Secretariat. He majored in Classics and obtained his BA degree in 1953. His studies continued at Princeton, where he obtained his MA in 1955 and his PhD in 1958, and was appointed Assistant to the Director by Professor Karl Erik Sjoquist, the Director of the Princeton excavations in Sicily. In the course of his studies and research, Kenan Erim had become fascinated by the sculptures attributed to a group of artists hailing from the ancient Graeco-Roman city of Aphrodisias, and in 1961 he organized his own expedition to explore and excavate the site. He has been Director of Excavations at Aphrodisias ever since. He is also Professor of

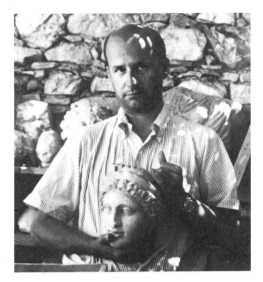

Classics at New York University, and divides his time between researching and teaching there, lecturing at Institutions throughout North America and in Europe, writing and publishing, and excavating each summer at Aphrodisias, where the continuing discoveries of superb sculpture, and remarkable monuments and architectural complexes reinforce his passionate and dedicated devotion to the site. His accomplishments have generated international interest and respect and he is the recipient of many honours and awards. Most recent among these is the Liberty Medal Award of New York City, which was presented on July 4th 1986 to him as one of a select number of distinguished immigrants to the United States of America, in recognition of their outstanding cultural and intellectual contributions to their adopted country.

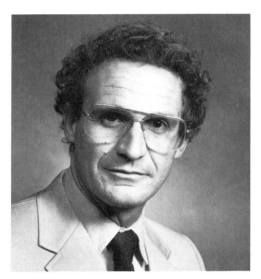

Jonathan S. Blair

From his days as a student in the United States of America, Jonathan Blair has been fascinated by history in general and archaeology in particular, although he began his career as a photographer in a different field entirely: astronomy. After leaving the Rochester Institute of Technology with a BS in Photographic Illustration he was taken on by the National Geographic Magazine and, in the early 1960s, one of his assignments took him to Aphrodisias. In those early days he found the site almost empty except for a few Turkish farmers, and felt as if he had travelled back in time, leaving the twentieth century far behind. His powerful first impressions of Aphrodisias, seeing it as it had come down through the ages, have remained with him. In his own words: "A lasting bond was to develop — and I continue to shoot at the site some twenty years after that first mystifying day."

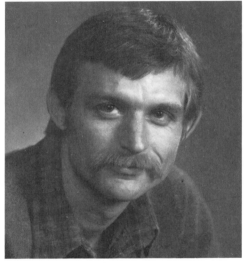

David L. Brill

David Brill was born in the United States of America in 1949 and has worked as a freelance photographer with the National Geographic Magazine since 1971, as well as following a successful career with advertising and commercial photographic work. The National Geographic Magazine has published his photographs in more than ten major articles, among which the excavations at Aphrodisias feature prominently. While at the site he was fascinated by the effects of light on statues and sculptural fragments, and found he could sense shapes and details that ordinary light seemed unable to reveal. This led him to develop techniques that would reveal the character and expression of his sculptural subjects — techniques that frequently involved shooting at night with multiple artificial light sources, but to the success of which this book bears ample witness.

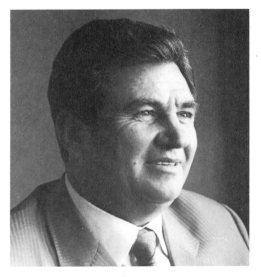

M. Ali Döğenci

Born in 1932, M. Ali Döğenci grew up and was educated in Bursa, Turkey, and began his photographic career there, before moving to Ankara to work as a freelance newspaper photographer. His specialization in archaeological photography began in 1958, when he was made responsible for the photographic laboratories of Ankara University's Archaeological Institute (Dil Tarih Coğrafya Fakültesi). Since then he has participated in many archaeological excavations conducted by the University, including those at Bayraklı, Çandarlı and Van (Adilcevaz). Between 1968 and 1984 he was the chief photographer of the Turkish Historical Society (Türk Tarih Kurumu) and supervised its photographic laboratory. In that capacity he continued to participate in many archaeological excavations, among them Erythrae (Ildırı), Maşat and Karahöyük (Konya). He has been a regular photographer with the Aphrodisias project since the 1960s.